Complete Hatha Yoga

Complete Hatha Yoga

Kevin and Venika Kingsland

Arco Publishing, Inc.
New York

Published by Arco Publishing, Inc.
215 Park Avenue South, New York, N.Y. 10003

Library of Congress Cataloging in Publication Data

Kingsland, Kevin.
   Complete hatha yoga.

   Bibliography: p.184
   Includes index.
   1. Yoga, Hatha.   I. Kingsland, Venika.   II. Title.
RA781.7.K54   1982   613.7'046   82-11586
ISBN 0-668-05559-6 (Cloth Edition)
ISBN 0-668-05561-8 (Paper Edition)

Printed in the United States of America

10   9   8   7   6   5   4   3   2   1

Contents

	page
Preface	7
Introduction	8

1 The Meaning of Yoga — 10
An absolute and a practical definition of yoga · The branches of yoga and the human personality—Karma Yoga · Hatha Yoga · Jnana Yoga · Bhakti Yoga · Mantra Yoga · Raja Yoga · Tantra Yoga · Ashtanga Yoga · A short history of yoga · A word on Sanskrit

2 The Stages of Yoga — 23
Asserting self-control—Yama · Observing and applying oneself—Niyama · Physical and mental exercise—Asana · Expanding ones energy—Pranayama · Sublimating and directing psychic energy—Pratyhara · Psychology of fixing the mind—Dharana · Psychology and philosophy of suggestion—Dhyana · Evolving awareness from individual to universal consciousness—Samadhi

3 Yama and Niyama—the Entrance Qualifications for Yoga — 28
Ahimsa · Satya · Asteya · Brahmacharya · Aparigraha · Saucha · Santosha · Tapasya · Svadhiyaya · Ishvarapranidhanani

4 The Chakra System I — 34
The traditional system · The spinal cord · The autonomic nervous system · the sympathetic division · the parasympathetic division · The brain · Reticular formation · The hypothalamus · The ventricles and cerebrospinal fluid · The cerebral cortex · Brain waves

5 The Chakra System II — 51
The endocrine system · The pineal · The pituitary · The thyroid · The thymus · The pancreas · The adrenals · The gonads

6 Akash and Prana — 64
Kumbhak and Prana · The circulatory system—the heart · control of heart rate · blood · The lymphatic and immune system · The respiratory system—nasal sinuses · the lungs and their capacity · control of respiration

7 Preparation for Yoga — 76
Preparing your mind · Environmental considerations · Timing · Preparing the body inside and out · Sankalpa · Composure

8 The Surya Namaskar   **81**
Method · Effects · Symbolism and mantras

9 Asanas   **88**
Asanas and psychosomatic tensions · Reasons for practising asanas · The order of an asana programme · Sukhasana · Vajrasana · Bhadrasana · Siddhasana · Padmasana · Sirshasana · Sarvangasana · Matsyasana · Gomukhasana · Paschimotanasana · Janusirasana · Bhujangasana · Salabhasana · Bhujangendrasana · Dhanurasana · Halasana · Suptavajrasana · Eka Pada Rajakapotasana · Chakrasana · Ushtrasana · Matsyendrasana · Ardha Matsyendrasana · Trikonasana · Chandrasana · Padhastasana · Garud-hasana · Natarajasana · Angusthasana · Eka Pada Angusthasana · Kaka-sana · Vatnyasana · Virabhadrasana · Anjaneyasana · Krounchasana · Simbhasana · Uttitha Kummerasana · Eye exercises

10 Mudras   **128**
Brahmas Mudra · Yoga Mudra · Mahabandha · Maha Mudra · Yoni Mudra · Aswini Mudra · Khechari Mudra · Bhoomi Sparsh Mudra · Jnana Mudra

11 Bandhas   **135**
Mulabandha · Uddiyanabandha · Jalandharabandha · Nadabandha · Brahmabandha · Jhivabandha · Viparitakarni

12 Pranayama   **140**
The order of practising Pranayama · Simple Pranayama · Suryabhedana · Ujjayi · Sitkari · Sitali · Bhastrika · Bhramari · Murccha

13 Kriyas   **147**
Dhauti · Basti · Nauli · Neti · Kapalbhati · Tratakam

14 Relaxation   **153**
The importance of relaxation · Shavasana · Yoga Nidra · Pratyhara

15 Tratakam   **159**
The power of the gaze · Simple Tratakam · Nasagra Drishti · Bhrumadhya Drishti

16 Meditation   **163**
The stages of meditation · Practical technique

17 The Importance of Food   **167**
Suitable food · Fasting

18 Some Considerations   **169**
Questions to be considered before starting yoga practice · How to test your teacher · Assessing your progress in yoga

19 Yoga in Everyday Life   **172**

References 175   **Glossary** 177   **Further Reading** 184

Acknowledgments 186   **Index** 187

Preface

The need for this book arose from our teaching at the Centre for Human Communication. Over the last twelve years we have taken many students through a wide range of practical, theoretical and professional courses in yoga subjects. Unfortunately there did not seem to be any books which could satisfy our need for a basically practical Hatha Yoga text which related intelligently to modern scientific knowledge. Most previous books were either clouded in unnecessary and obscure traditional yoga terminology or were watered-down modern journalistic fabrication. In any case the books which did not ring with a lack of both understanding and practical experience of yoga were very rare and most difficult to obtain.

K. and V.K.
Centre for Human Communication
Davidsonville, Maryland

Introduction

It is not the chaos and disorderliness of the world which is the cause of restlessness, dissension and disharmony, and hot and cold war, but the lack of unity which causes all the conflicting challenges around and within us.

Unity means yoga and yoga means unity, and this unity cannot be created but should be experienced within our inner self. He who has not experienced this inner unity cannot create unity outside, although he may talk throughout his life on the subject. He who has no confidence within himself but tries to find confidence and unity through others is doomed to failure. Thus yoga presents unity in all phases of reality. The matter becomes perfect when its unity is realised in the form of electricity. The electricity becomes perfect when its unity is realised in the form of life and the various forms of energy. The life becomes perfect when the universe of sensation and mentation comes into evolution. The universe of sensation becomes perfect when it is evolved in the form of absolute and eternal consciousness, which is the basic foundation of the entire universe in all its phases. To realise this thread of unity, yoga philosophy presents the following stepping stones.

1 HATHA YOGA Through hatha yoga one makes the body ready, like a cosmic television or radio, to receive and transmit waves of energy from the universe and to the universe. We live in the ocean of energy as fish live in the ocean of water. The operation of energy is two-fold, the first part being sent through a network of wires, and the second without wires, in the form of radio waves. Hatha yoga prepares our body for both purposes. The body finds integrity and harmony as each organ and system co-operates with other organs and systems through association fibres within the brain. This is like the operation of electricity through wires. Hatha yoga also prepares this body to receive vibration from other solar systems and planets and to transmit waves back to them like radio waves. Thus it removes feelings of loneliness and isolation. This process of coming into contact with the entire universe by means of energy is called *pranayama*.

2 MANTRA YOGA Mantra yoga is the direction of the psychodynamics, or

the movement of the individual mind, from the individual existence to the cosmic existence.

3 LAYA YOGA Laya yoga is the transmission of individual mental energy into cosmic energy. It is the absorption and submergence of individual existence in cosmic existence. In religious language it is the submergence of the individual soul into godhood.

4 RAJA YOGA Raja yoga is the discovery of the thread of unity running through all multiplicity.

5 INTEGRAL YOGA Integral yoga is the application of raja yoga to bring all manifestation of reality into togetherness.

Hatha yoga is the basic foundation of all yoga, because without body nothing can be accomplished. Although there are three types of meditation—relative, transcendental and supratranscendental, they all depend on the integrity of body. It is hatha yoga which prepares the body for the three types of meditation. hatha contains two words—*ha* and *tha*. *Ha* means the sun and *tha* means the moon in Sanskrit; *ha* the supreme self and *tha* the individual self; *ha* the noumenon and *tha* the phenomenon; *ha* the unity and *tha* the multiplicity. Thus the meeting or union of the *ha* and *tha* is called hatha yoga which begins from the discipline of the body and ends in the experience of the Self— one-without-a-second, or double.

At present there is a tremendous interest in yoga and its various techniques which has led to a flood of books on the subject. Why should there be any new addition to this flood? The answer lies in the simple and practical approach of Kevin and Venika Kingsland, an approach which is most refreshing in the current flood. What has not been explained in recent times is the practical application of yoga in our daily life as a way of understanding ourselves and the universe around us, and of experiencing the unity and harmony which is the need of our time. This is what the Kingslands' book does and I hope its readers will enjoy and benefit immensely from it.

RAMAMURTI S MISHRA MD

1 The Meaning of Yoga

Yoga is now an everyday word in the West. Yoga programmes appear on television while the glossy magazines are filled with pages of yoga-related literature and interviews with famous people who have 'taken up' yoga. In England alone, at least 100,000 people are known to attend regular classes in yoga. During the last two or three years over 500 yoga teachers have appeared, as from nowhere, to instruct and guide the needy.

There are those who believe that to practise yoga means 'legs up, head down and a few vegetables a day'. Some think erroneously that yoga is a kind of oriental religion. But even so, it is likely that today the average westerner will know more about yoga than his Indian counterpart. Although yoga has been ascribed to India it did not originate there.

There are two important definitions of yoga: it can be seen either as a state or as a process—the absolute and the practical. The word *yoga* comes from a root word *yug* meaning 'to unite'. This state of unity does not mean there is any unity between a lower and a higher Self. It does not refer to the Self at all, for there is only one Self—no one has ever experienced two selves. It is possible to experience two persons or two minds or any amount of 'things', but the Self is not a 'thing'. Anything that can be experienced physically, mentally or emotionally, is the object of experience as distinct from the subject, or Self, who does the experiencing. The Self is like light. Light itself is never seen, but only the objects which it illuminates. In a room it is the walls and furniture that are seen, not light. In a lamp, it is the glass bulb and filament that are seen. You may think you see a beam of light shining through a darkened room, but it is the dust in the atmosphere that you see, not the light. In the same way it is through consciousness, Self, that we experience the universe. Consciousness itself is never seen, but its existence is known about by the things it illuminates. It is itself a nothing.

Another word for nothing is 'space'. It is impossible to say what space is, although it is easy to say what it is not. Space is not the atmosphere in which we live. If we consider a tiny volume of the so-called space in a room this point will be made clear.

There is a simple kind of camera called a pin-hole camera. It does not have a lens but light enters it through a small hole about the size of a pin prick. Light sufficient to photograph one end of our room passes through this point in 'space'. We could take countless photographs of the room in as great a detail as we wished by rotating the camera about this point in all directions. We could, of course, remove all the light by placing a black box around our point in space and remove the air and dust particles by creating a vacuum inside. Remember, a perfect vacuum has still not been attained in any scientific laboratory, even though vacuums may be created which have less material in them than deep 'space' has. Again, we could place a radio or television at that point in space and tune in to countless programmes which come not only from broadcasting stations all over the earth but from innumerable radio sources in outer space. Cosmic particles and waves continually pass through our point. We could place a compass at our point and it would indicate the presence of a magnetic field and of electric charges, ever changing as the environment modifies. It would be possible to reduce the electromagnetic material in our space by shielding it with copper or iron. (This arrangement is called a Faraday cage, after Michael Faraday who used it in his experiments during the last century.) Dr Puharich[1] has carried out some very interesting experiments placing people inside Faraday cages. He found that as the subjects were better and better shielded from the earth's electromagnetism, they became more and more psychic. It would seem that what is called a 'psiplasma field' also fills our space. To complete the picture, gravity waves are passing through our space all the time.

Having illustrated that what we commonly think of as space is not space at all, it becomes evident that it is a very elusive entity indeed. Space cannot be felt or tasted, it is not possible to smell it or hear it and it cannot be seen. It is impossible to conceptualise except negatively and it cannot even be imagined. This tempts us to conclude that space does not exist, but then again that is precisely what nothing is—something which does not exist. It is almost like a riddle: 'What exists yet does not exist?' The answer is 'space'. (The space considered here should not be confused with the time-space continuum of physics which affects matter and is itself affected by matter.)

Space itself cannot be affected. It is transcendental. It cannot be altered in any way. It is changeless, eternal, omnipresent. This is what the ancient researchers—'rishis'—called Brahman. What is called space is identical to Self. Here we are not talking about the arbitrary collection of things which we identify with and label 'me'. This is our ego, not our Self. Self is sometimes described as I 'am' as against the experience 'I am this' or 'I am that'. The description, 'I am myself no thing' is not a statement of humility, but a cosmic truth.

Space cannot be divided; and that is just what 'individual' means. There is only one individual; there is only one Self. Space, however, can appear to be divided when, through light, objects are manifested. But we know through the experimental investigations of modern scientists that even the smallest particle, such as an electron, is omnipresent. That is, matter is not discrete; it does not have a surface, like a billiard ball seems to have, but spreads out to infinity. It is the nature of our perception that gives us the impression that objects have edges and are separate. Nothing in the universe is separate; all is one in an ocean of vibration and music. The rishis called the state of realising this oneness Yoga and the state of apparent differentiation Maya.

The fundamental capacity which the Self has is the power to identify. When we are in a room which is pitch dark we are not able to differentiate anything. When electrical light is switched on we can clearly see that the room is filled with objects, but what we see depends entirely on what kind of light we are using. If we looked at the room through the eyes of an owl or a bee we would experience it quite differently. The owl sees infra-red light, which we do not, so it can spot a mouse on a moonless, unlighted night. Photographs of cars and other objects can be taken *after* they have been removed from a position they were formerly occupying by an infra-red camera. If we could see infra-red we would be able to see the diseased areas in people's bodies, as the infra-red light given off from a person's body depends on the flow of blood and fluids beneath the skin. Diseased areas are typically deprived of nourishment and blood supply and so show up as cold areas in the body. The bee sees ultra-violet light, and its universe is quite different again.

Our perceptual awareness provides one way of looking at the universe. It is not 'wrong', but simply partial. What we experience is an illusion not necessarily a delusion. When white light is passed through coloured film it produces a picture on a screen. The colours on the screen are not 'added' to the white light but are rather what is left after the film has 'subtracted' the remaining light. What we experience is not unreal as such, it is simply only a part of reality. Our problem is that we tend to experience some small fragment of the universe of vibration and believe that it is the whole of reality.

'Whole' comes from an old Anglo-Saxon word *hal* from which we have also derived 'holy' and 'health'. This complete and whole state is a state in which no separation or change is experienced. Tension and stress depend upon separation and differentiation, and therefore cannot exist in the state of Yoga. In the state of Yoga no thing, no separation, is experienced. The idea of unification refers not to the Self, for it cannot be divided, but to the universe of experience. The apparently divided universe is arbitrarily labeled 'me' and 'not me'. These labels are not permanent but change with a process which is called 'learning' or 'personal growth'. Moreover, these labels are quite distinct for different personalities. Personality is a phenomenon of the universe and so it is appropriate to talk about different personalities. Ultimately we know that there is no such distinction. For a moment, however, we are identifying with the universe of relativity.

The word 'person' comes from *persona* meaning a 'mask' of the kind an actor puts on to play a role. The personality changes with every situation. A person will describe himself in the way he experiences himself, while his friends will describe him as they experience him. At work a person may play the role of an efficient, hardheaded business man; at home he may play the role of a husband and a father; and with old school friends he may play the fool. The person may not notice that he is playing many roles, but when by chance he finds himself in the simultaneous company of his wife, children, old school friends and business colleagues he may find it acutely embarrassing, not knowing which role to play.

Personality can thus be harmonious or disharmonious. The person can be more or less healthy, whole, or diseased. The disease is called physical, mental or spiritual according to the person who is diagnosing it. Most people suffer from disease at some time. Today the stress diseases are becoming more and more common, and the big killers, such as arterio sclerosis, cancer, coronary thrombosis, are almost certainly manifestations of increasing psychosomatic stress. About half the hospital beds in Britain are given over to mental patients, while something like one in three of the general population is said to have a referable mental problem at some time during their life. The situation is not apparently improving at all. It is no comfort that per head of population one of the highest suicide rates is that amongst psychiatrists themselves.

The practice of yoga is any means, technique, exercise or process by which the absolute state of Yoga can be realised. This is a very wide and comprehensive definition. Indeed, yoga practice is accurately described as the 'positive half of life'. Many people are practising yoga and do not know it. Yoga is for all.

The Branches of Yoga and Human Personality

There is only one starting point for any of us in our attempt to attain self-realisation or state of Yoga. It is the point at which we are here and now; the point with which we identify. Every person is unique, no less than every snow-flake, but if we ask people to describe who they think they are we may nevertheless discover a general group of patterns which can be used to classify the person in a general way.

Personality descriptions can be categorised to eight major levels of personal identification. There are similarly about eight basic starting points in yoga practice, some of which will be more suitable for one kind of personality than another. These are sometimes called the branches of yoga.

Karma Yoga

The first kind of personality is that of the man of action. Characteristically this person identifies strongly with his physical body and feels that life is to be lived energetically and intensely. He gets bored if nothing is happening in an outward way. He is not interested in discussion or reading, he must manipulate the concrete world. Usually this person places his security in his physical health and the branch of Yoga which suits his personality is Karma Yoga.

Karma Yoga is the yoga of action. It is the fulfilment of Self through doing things; the attainment of Yoga by doing what you believe it is right to do. People practising Karma Yoga are discovered cleaning up polluted sites, working in voluntary organisations to help the underprivileged, building new communities and generally 'doing their thing'.

What we do depends upon what we feel and think. What we feel and think depends upon what we identify with, which in turn depends upon what we have learned about. We have no problems connected with what we have learned fully—complete knowledge is identical to Yoga—it is what we partially know

13

that causes us all sorts of problems. Whatever we know completely, we do not have to remember. Driving a car or playing the piano are skills which do not require remembering, only directing. What we have hardly learned at all, we do not remember at all. We may remember a telephone number just long enough to dial it and then forget it. Each time we need to call that same number we have to look it up, thus repeating the learning process over and over again until we can clearly remember the number and no longer need to look it up. It is the same in life. Situations we have not learned from we are inclined to repeat again and again, and if we do not learn from our mistakes the lessons tend to get tougher. This process is called karma.

When we have partially learned something then it may be stored in our long-term memory. Unless we are aware of our long-term memory it can affect our whole lives. For example, the experiences of our childhood have played a large role in shaping the nature of our adult life. Hence it has been said that the child is father to the man. This kind of effect is sometimes called 'conditioning'. In Yoga these memory traces are called samskaras. Most people have never bothered or thought anything about the samskaras that influence our behaviour. We carry on life ignorant of the limitations that we are putting on ourselves. Like the caterpillar which builds its own prison, we encage ourselves in the influences of our own education and social contacts. Very few of us are self-starters, initiating our own lives and becoming our own leaders. We remain the puppets of our own self-limitations.

Karma Yoga is precisely the process of taking life in our own hands and getting on with it. By conscious, self-initiated action we fulfil and transcend our karma to obtain the highest state of Yoga.

Hatha Yoga

The next type of person does not identify so completely with the body. He feels that life is something more, rather like the electricity manifesting through a light bulb. He identifies with some kind of vital energy. His security is largely invested in friends as he feels that whilst the body may become diseased or maimed, if you have friends to help you then all will be well. For this person life is experienced as a series of ups and downs. One moment he feels optimistic and full of energy, the next moment he feels depressed and depleted. His life is confused.

Hatha Yoga is a discipline for all who are fed up with the pendulum swings of life. Whilst the darkest hours may be just before dawn, tomorrow is another day which also has a night! Life is the repetition of day and night, sun and moon. *Ha* means 'sun' and *tha* means 'moon'. Hatha Yoga is the method by which the opposites of life may be transcended and a singleness of mind and consistency of action may be attained.

This book is largely about Hatha Yoga so a special description is unnecessary here, but briefly it is an integrated system of personal development by which the vicissitudes of life can be transcended, psychosomatic tensions can be removed

14

and personal horizons can be extended. Through overcoming the constant flux of life, the unchanging, radiant Self may shine through as a light to guide all people out of the darkness of confusion.

Jnana Yoga

The third type of person is not particularly interested in action or physical exercises, considering both somewhat below him. This is the intellectual who approaches life through knowledge. He believes that life is to be experienced and that change and novelty are the essence of life. He tends to place his security in his ability to adapt to any situation.

It is well known that the feline species is depleted as the result of its own curiosity. Discrimination is required, and Jnana Yoga is a means by which discrimination may be nourished through clearly distinguishing various kinds of experience. The individual who does not know what is real and what is not real, who cannot differentiate the temporal from the eternal, who cannot tell what is right or wrong in a given situation, is liable to base his life on false assumptions. This may result in building a house on sand, whereas if the house of our life is constructed on a firm foundation of rock it will not be undermined by the environmental conditions.

Many a basically positive person has lacked the power of discrimination—called viveka in Sanskrit. The result for these deluded people has not been a Jacob's ladder, which they falsely believed led up to heaven, but a stairway to hell constructed by their own good intentions. It is not sufficient to have a good intellect. A half-sharp intellect may simply cut the owner, whereas a razor-sharp intellect can keenly cut through any Gordian knot which might prevent others becoming the master of themselves.

Jnana Yoga is the yoga of knowledge. The root word *jna* is seen in 'gno' in gnosis and 'kno' in knowledge. It is not the mere study of information, but the process of discriminating between the real Self and the objects of experience. The person who has achieved this realisation is called a jnani.

Many people who are classed as intellectuals do not really have very good intellects. They are deeply involved in intellectual pursuits because they have not yet fully understood the nature of the intellect. The intellect is a cutting instrument which divides up the universe. Just as light illuminates an object, showing one side clearly and throwing the other side into shadow, so the intellect illuminates one point at the expense of another. The creation of the intellect is logic. There are many kinds of logic but the most frequently used is the logic of cause and effect. To justify this logic a higher logic is required, and a higher logic again is required to produce that and so on. Logic is one tool by which information may be manipulated but it is not the only tool.

The intellectual must clearly see reality and initially examine the Self by the light of the intellect. It is rather like holding up a lamp to look at the sun. Using logical processes he decides that the moon is in fact far more important than the sun, because at night we need the light more. Much of science and particularly

15

the main schools of western psychology have been examining the universe intellectually. For a long time subjects such as consciousness and love have largely been ignored in favour of other areas which are easier for the intellectual to study.

Jnana Yoga, then, is the process of cutting through all life's alternative games with the aim of seeking first the Self, the kingdom of Heaven. The person who applies his intellect to undisciplined experience is merely diffusing his psychic energy. It is like the professor who was being ferried across a lake. He asked the ferryman whether he had ever studied philosophy, to which the ferryman replied, 'No, I never did nothing like that'. The professor reprimanded the fellow saying, 'Have you never studied grammar? Half your life has been wasted'. The ferryman said nothing, but soon a storm blew up and the boat started sinking in the water. The ferryman asked the professor 'Have you ever studied swimming? No? Then your whole life has been wasted because we are sinking'.

Self cannot be known through books or study. The *Bhagavad Gita* asks 'What use is a pond where everywhere is flood?'[2] Books are of like use to the jnani. Self, being the observer, is not known as it is the knower. Whilst the whole universe can potentially be known, the Self is that which cannot be known. It is itself knowledge. Hence the statement: 'It is not what you know that is important. It is knowing what you do not know that is important.' The essence of Jnana Yoga is summed up in the *Kenopanishad*[3]: 'He who thinks he knows, knows not. He who knows he knows not, really knows.'

Bhakti Yoga

The next type of person identifies with the things he possesses; that which he says is 'mine'. Other people with inflated egos are a particular threat to him, and much of his energy goes into asserting himself and dominating, if possible, other people. If he is outwardly inclined then he wants a lot of money, if he is inwardly inclined he may set himself up as a guru and acquire many students and disciples. This is the business tycoon who through his acquisitive aggressiveness gains great prestige and has people attending him, pandering to his inflated ego image. If he is successful he will very likely have his name on the lips of millions of people as a brand name or perhaps a star or, most cunningly, as a spiritual leader.

Bhakti Yoga is the method of transcending the ego by devoted service. The person who has a need to assert himself is basically insecure. The strong ego is so confident that it does not have to compensate by over-asserting itself. Only the truly self-disciplined can serve without being servile. Only the real teacher can wash the feet of his disciples and be a living example of service. The man who has mastered his ego may lay it aside in the cause of greater good. The great Bhakti Yogi may even lay down his life for his fellow men. He does it joyfully through strength, for though he may be crucified by others, he is in absolute control of his own universe. The great Bhakti yogi does not need to be proclaimed king. He who would be first in the eyes of society may be last in the realisation that the ego is but one tool in the cosmic workshop, and as such is no better and no worse than any other, is the perfect goal of Bhakti Yoga. The Bhakti yogi serves the universe without thought of any personal gain. He gives service simply, because love overwhelms the personality and he cannot help but serve. He helps the needy, heals the sick, visits the lonely and aged. The labour of Bhakti Yoga is carried out in love, and there are no regrets or personal desires.

The Bhakti yogi is not a do-gooder, for the do-gooder is basically an egotist. What we do is the exact result of what we are as a person. The tree is known by its fruits; thus if we are good then everything we do has good results. No one is qualified in reality to judge another. However, the actions of a person may be judged. If a man says he loves God but hates people then he is deluded. First we have to love other people, then we are able to completely love ourselves and only then can we truly love God.

The person who believes that he is serving God is really on what has come to be known, correctly, in contemporary language as a 'big ego trip'. God does not need any mortal help. If he does then he is holding down a job under false pretences. The person who thinks that he alone is the incarnation of God is also on an ego trip. There is only one Self and it manifests through all things. There is no room for one-upmanship. The hand cannot say to the foot that because it is not the hand it is of less use. Any person who feels superior to others is spiritually quite mistaken. The practice of Bhakti Yoga is the way of mastering the ego and discovering that all is Self.

Mantra Yoga

The fifth type of personality is that of the thinker. He has precise and rather fixed ideas about life. He is a natural conservative and will do anything to keep the peace. He is usually tolerant of other people's ideas, but is not truly prepared to consider them and is the victim of his own semantic reactions. He feels that he more or less understands the universe and that he simply has to tidy up his ideas a little to complete the picture. He places his security in some figure of authority. He typically believes in some gospel truth, be it the written word of a religious book or the latest statements in a respected scientific journal. He tends to idealise the universe and if, for example, his wife were to leave him for another man he would feel shocked and be unable to understand why she did it, believing himself to have been a loving husband and a good, loyal provider. The family is very important to him and much of his life is centred around it. He thinks carefully about life and typically keeps himself well-informed by fully reading the newspapers. He may be aware that the earth is running out of resources, polluting itself and rapidly becoming overpopulated, but he is confident that 'they' will do something about it. 'They' always have, so he is not too worried and need not make any great personal effort, although if called upon he will, of course, do his bit. He cannot understand the emotionality of others, but

17

not everyone can be expected to be as rational and cool headed as he is.

This person's fixed ideas prevent him from growing and passing beyond thinking to the direct experience of Self. Mantra Yoga is a method by which he may follow certain paths of reasoning which lead to greater insights. Through specific techniques he is enabled to lay aside his thinking, which is merely the manipulation of memory traces, and through perfect inner silence realise the Self.

Usually this person fails to perceive that the outside authority which he recognises is an authority only because he judges it one and labels it so. In order to realise that the Self is the author of all things he has to discover his inner authority. Mantra Yoga is the method of transcending all thoughts and concepts to experience the undefinable, inconceivable reality—the Self—by stopping all thinking. Very few people can stop their thinking at will. Most people have very little control over their thoughts and find that they come into their mind every few seconds whether they like it or not. *Man* comes from a word meaning 'thought', and *tra* stems from a word indicating 'protection'. A little more will be written about Mantra in the chapter on meditation.

Raja Yoga

There is a type of person who finds it very difficult to describe who they think they are. Such people feel part of some greater whole but are not quite sure what. They may well give up mundane existence in order to travel the world in search of a teacher who can help them discover their true selves. They put their trust in something greater than themselves.

These people are naturally contemplative and enjoy beautiful surroundings and sensitive communication. They do not really like the nasty, insensitive world, and dream of escaping to a Shangri-la. Raja Yoga is a way of discovering that there is no real distinction between individual and cosmic Self. There is only one Self and that I am. I am not this 'I am' which refers to my ego image, I am that 'I am', which is the real Self. *I am that I am.*

Raja Yoga is the supreme yoga, the king of methods, by which one directly experiences the Self through laying aside all else. It requires vast concentration power and provides great inner direction, enabling the Raja yogi to live in the midst of confusion and ignorance and yet be untouched by it. The Raja yogi may be in the world, but he is not of it. He is like the famous lotus flower, which springs from the mud of ignorance and rests untouched on the waters of the world.

Tantra Yoga

There is a particular kind of person who lives in a great awareness of the creative power of the imagination. By the word imagination a very real and powerful aspect of the universe is indicated. The word imagination has of late been held in low esteem in the West as a result of being confused with the imaginary. Hallucination, delusion and day-dreaming have been considered the essence of imagination, and indeed these are the realms of this seventh personality when it chooses escapism rather than facing up to the world. This person is to be found 'stoned' under the chemical effects of lysergic acid, mescalin or psylocibin.

The biological effect of hallucinogenic drugs is to disinhibit the firing of brain cells. Instead of their normal moderate activity, the neurons are thrown into a highly excited state in which anything can happen. In records of the electrical activity of epileptic brains during *grand mal,* and deliberately controlled studies of yogis raising the Kundalini Shakti, we see similar patterns.

The brain, like a government, is basically an inhibitory mechanism, stopping and slowing natural progress. We all have enormous creative ability and the potential to learn thoroughly at a very fast rate if it can only be released. In Bulgaria[4] people are taught how to relax, disinhibit, and learn new skills such as a foreign language in a few weeks. Modern man is rather like the totally primitive tribe who had had no contact with civilisation when they discovered an undamaged Land-Rover abandoned by an expedition in the middle of their territory. First of all they played with it, until a genius discovered that if a rope was tied to the front bumper, it could be pulled along by several men and used as a sledge to move things. Then the handbrake was discovered. When it was released far fewer men were required to move the vehicle and this was a cause for great celebrations. In a similar way, man is about to discover the handbrake on his mind.

This seventh personality places his security on his own ability to create a solution to any problem that might arise through use of his imagination. The imagination may be limited at first but it can be expanded. The imagination has put man on the moon. It is a very powerful force; for example, under hypnosis a subject may imagine a pencil to be a red-hot poker and will come up in a blister if he is touched with it. The imagination can cure 'incurable' diseases, or inspire vast groups of people to go to war or build a new society. The imagination can kill and it can give birth. It can ignite the world with new ideas which may spread like wildfire. It can also imprison the personality, like a chicken in an imaginary shell from which it cannot escape.

Tan means 'to spread' and *tra* indicates the power of the imagination to 'save' the personality from delusion. Tantra is a method of experimentation and practice to expand the imagination, so that the universe may be discovered to be nothing but the weaving of the cosmic imagination. The universe of experience is the result of continuous imaginations, just as the glowing embers in a log fire may suggest enchanted worlds and fascinating stories. It is easy to sit staring into the cosmic fire as though in a trance. For those who are not awake to themselves the practices of Tantra Yoga may appear ritualistic or dangerous. If we did not understand the nature of fire, the collecting of dry sticks and then laying them in a prescribed manner with dried leaves or paper at the centre would be ritualistic. The flint and iron we strike one upon the other in the way we have been instructed would be ritual instruments—but only because we lack understanding. After applied practice we may transcend the ritual.

The power of the universe which manifests through the imagination is called Shakti. Energy in its potential state is often associated with a spiral form, such as that described by the path of earth through space. DNA, which holds the power to direct and create entire organisms such as the human body, is in the form of a spiral. The Sanskrit word for spiral is Kundali and Kundalini is the embodiment of this spiral energy. The universe of energy is sometimes called 'mother nature', and this is the essence of Shakti. When the universe of power and energy is called Shakti, the Self is referred to as Shiva. Shiva and Shakti are considered two aspects of a whole and are often imagined as cosmic male and female. The female, Shakti, is active, and thus is portrayed on top of Shiva and the empirical universe is seen to be the intercourse between Consciousness and Energy.

Energy exists only because of a differentiation between the observer and the thing observed, and as long as there appears to be a separation between Self and non-Self, the universe of energy will manifest. The tendency to remove separation is called love. Love is the energy of unification, which, at a basic level, is sexual and individual energy, and is symbolised by the coiled serpent which represents Kundalini. It is only the partially in love, however, that experience the sexual drive, for when no separation is experienced between people no energy, and thus no sex drive, exists. The sexual act is the building up of tensions until male and female—positive and negative—energies balance, and in the neutralisation the experience of non-separation—union—is attained. The bliss of sexual orgasm is the experience of being. Self is described as Satchitananda and is existence, consciousness, bliss. The yogi in union with Self is experiencing a cosmic orgasm. At the other end of the scale the sneeze is also an orgasm, as for a split second there is no experience but that of being.

The essence of yoga practice is the removal of separation. Separation is epitomised in Tantra Yoga as male and female energies. However the separation is within oneself, and it is a mistake to project it outside. It is quite possible to misunderstand Tantra Yoga by materialising the Tantric practices. One must realise that further involution with matter by allowing an undisciplined imagination to stir up basic energies is the opposite practice to that of Tantra Yoga. Through mastery of Tantra Yoga separation disappears and the universe appears to dissolve. This is called Laya in Sanskrit.

Ashtanga Yoga

The final group of people is not easily classified. They seem to be all-rounders who do not identify with anything in particular. They understand the importance of material things such as food, money and machines and can use them well when required, but they are not ruled by them. Their approach to life is so widely based that they do not place their security in anything, for they feel no need of security. They are independent but not isolated; psychologically alone but not lonely. They understand that the universe is one of change in which nothing exists for ever. For them nothing is more important than that they should do what is right at the time Happiness and fulfilment are their reasons for living, and they have no regrets and no anxieties. Wherever they find themselves they are basically content, although this does not imply that they lack ambition. Indeed their ambition may be supreme—to manifest the Self perfectly.

The kind of yoga these people practise is called Ashtanga Yoga. *Asht* means 'eight' and *anga* means 'limbs'. Thus Ashtanga is a way of life which involves the entire spectrum of personality. It is the practice of all the branches of yoga at once.

A further branch of yoga—new compared to the methods described above—is called Catering Yoga. This has sprung up fairly recently and is basically a form of entertainment. It is designed for people who wish to satisfy their need to be doing something positive about their own lives but are not actually prepared to make any fundamental changes in their way of life. It has been fabricated from various branches of yoga and is rather like a soup made from a soup from a chicken—very watered down and with little nutrition left in it. As many people today have lost their taste buds and cannot easily distinguish between margarine and butter, hot air and cigarette smoke, hot water or tea, it is easy to understand that there is plenty of room for this branch of yoga.

The idea is that yoga should be made easy for people. It should be potted, condensed, simplified, translated and marketed, providing something for people to do and talk about as an alternative to a lot of other, more dubious, pursuits. Catering Yoga is basically a very positive movement, but unfortunately there are many who are jumping on to the yoga band-wagon and thus bringing yoga into disrepute. There are some people involved who are merely seeking to make money and others who are on a 'big ego trip'.

Economic considerations are not in themselves unyogic, for a yogi is a master of all things, money included. However, the point being made here is that there are many choices available in yoga and the potential student should be sure that he is practising the branch of yoga that best suits his needs. The yogi is the first to acknowledge the individual's freedom to choose any life style he wishes, but that freedom carries with it the total responsibility for all his actions.

A Short History of Yoga

Ancient Indian researchers were very exact in their measurement of time and space.[5] Whilst in the West many people still believed the world to have been created in about 4004 BC, the Indian had already obtained a highly realistic estimate of the age of the universe. The creation and destruction of the universe is said to be a breath of braham—the absolute Self. It is called a Kalpa and is 4,320,000,000 years long, an estimate which is closely comparable with modern scientific calculations. The Kalpa is divided into fourteen manvantara, which in turn are divided into seventy-one mahayuga, each lasting 4,320,000 years. The mahayuga is divided into four yugas known as Satya, Treeta, Dvapar and Kali.

There are short periods of transition between the eras which account for other-wise unaccounted time.

The roots of yoga can be traced back to the Satyayuga, the golden age of righteousness, when the Vedas, known as *Sruti*, and Upanishads were first revealed to man. The source of the Vedas may thus be attributed to a time in excess of 2 million years ago, although western researchers and westernised Indian scholars prefer to date them much later as they find it difficult to believe that man was intelligent before a sudden blossoming a few thousand years ago. The Satyayuga lasted about 1,728,000 years. The second age, called Treetayuga, lasted 1,296,000 years, and during this time the *Smriti* was compiled dealing with all aspects of social law and behaviour. The *puranas*, sacred Sanskrit poems, were composed to guide the people of the third age—Dvarparyuga—which lasted about 864,000 years. The present age is called the Kaliyuga and is the age of change. The Tantra and related works were, and still are, being written for this time which began about 5,000 years ago and will last 432,000 years.

The most exciting thing about traditional yoga is that it has been tried and tested over many thousands of years, in contrast to modern techniques—such as Thalidomide—which are often hardly tested at all. We know a great deal about ancient yoga, not only through the knowledge handed down by word of mouth but also from the original literature which still exists. The ancient writers wrote on palm leaves which had been chemically treated to withstand damp and resist fire. Today, these manuscripts can still be seen, although they are mostly preciously preserved from the public. But like the Dead-Sea Scrolls they remain as an original testimony of man's incredible history and it is hoped that the temples and individuals who possess these scripts will be motivated one day to avail them to qualified scientists for carbon dating and translation.

A Word on Sanskrit

Just as Italian is the language of music and Latin of science, so Sanskrit is the language of yoga. *Sanskrit* means 'mathematically and scientifically exact language'. Sanskrit words are used in this book and we believe that Sanskrit will be integrated into all world languages, especially English, during the next decades. Sanskrit is probably one of the easiest languages in the world to learn as the grammar is precise and written Sanskrit is perfectly phonetic. It is probable that most indo-aryan languages including English have their origins in a language similar to Vedic Sanskrit. The Sanskrit[6] alphabet is a logical array of vocal sounds and each letter is a basic root word. All Sanskrit words are built up from these basic phonemic blocks and thus every word reveals its own meaning like a formula. There are many reasons why we believe Sanskrit terms should be maintained in yoga practice, the least being the great semantic loss incurred through inadequate English equivalents. The introduction of Sanskrit terms in this book will lay a foundation for further study of more traditional and philosophical texts.

2 The Stages of Yoga

The state of Yoga cannot be fully realised whilst the individual identifies with the non-self, the manifested universe of vibration. That which a person identifies with is called his ego; it is everything which he labels 'me' and varies considerably from person to person. The ego structure reflects the nature of the universe just as a random sample of people interviewed for an opinion poll tends to reflect the attitudes and behaviour of the population as a whole. Different egos do not vary in their general structure, but are distinguished through varying degrees of emphasis on any one category of elements. For example, all people have some degree of physical identification or they would not be incarnated, but while some people are very highly identified with their body, believing that it is the essential person, others hardly identify with their body at all, and see it only as an instrument for manifesting consciousness.

There is one statement that is such an evident truth that it seems almost superfluous to state it: there is nothing easier to be than what you are already. The state of Yoga requires no effort to be realised, it requires a letting go of all effort. It is the continual effort to be something other than what we really are that is the cause of all our problems.

The image a man has of himself is called his ego. The image another man has of him is called his personality. Every person will have a unique image of any other man which will depend upon the ego of the person observing the man, and the role the man is playing in the situation concerned. There might be as many personality descriptions are there are observations. If a man's experience of himself matches the experience other people have of him, then he is said to see himself clearly. If, however, his ego image bares little resemblence to the way other people experience him, he is said to be deluded. The identification of the Self—the experiencer—with the non-self—the object of experience—is an illusion. The precise process of yoga is the removal of this illusion (Maya) through discriminating (viveka) clearly between Self and non-self.

The release from this illusion may be accomplished instantly, but most people refuse to let go without a fight. These are the people who diligently search the world in order to discover themselves and finally, after exhausting all other possibilities, realise that the one who was doing the searching was the one they were looking for, like the man who searches frantically for his glasses until, catching a glimpse of himself in a mirror, he realises that he is actually wearing them. The majority of people prefer the longer, harder way, just as a person will often prefer to make an extra journey rather than expend a little mental effort to check whether he has remembered everything clearly the first time.

It can seem a very difficult task to be yourself. To those who have already felt the death-pangs of their hopes and ideals the suggestion that there is a greater reality, a deeper purpose to life, sounds like every other overused slogan they have heard before. For those who are confused by conflicting statements, who are overpowered by the strong current of daily affairs, a step-by-step, fully testable, verifiable method has been designed to lead them back to Self. For those who cannot jump there is a step-ladder on which each experiental rung represents a stage of dehypnosis, enabling one to retrace creation back to Self.

The belief that certain objects of experience are in fact the Self, created the ego in the first place. As the caterpillar builds a cocoon around itself in order to be born again as a beautiful butterfly, so man cocoons himself with material ideas, thoughts and images engendered by his environment, education and social contacts and background. Unless a man clears his mind deliberately his whole life will be limited and conditioned by early suggestions. When we clear out a drawer that has accumulated things for years, we throw out layer after layer as we come to it. In clearing up our personality we do very much the same.

Having lived life without real direction for a very long time we are psychically dispersed and disordered. 'Discipline' comes from a word meaning 'to learn', and self-discipline is the process of optimising our learning. Our energy is dissipated over a lot of more or less irrelevant activities which are alternatives to self-discovery, and in order to learn the purpose of life and who we really are we must take a hold on ourself. The first stage of yoga experience, called *Yama*, involves just this. It is the firm determination to take the reins of our life in our hands and to guide our life along the path of self-discovery out of the quagmire of destructive instinctual forces (vitarka) which cloud our understanding.

Having decided to be the director of our own life rather than the proverbial straw blown about by the winds of the world, we have lighted a fire which is difficult to extinguish. The dross that is not the pure gold of Self will sooner or later be burned away, and the stages of psychological and spiritual growth follow naturally. There are definite restraints (yamas) which we place upon our behaviour as we manifest self-discipline, and there are likewise definite activities (niyamas) which we will encourage and nourish in ourselves. Niyama is the second stage of yoga in which we invoke the cosmic law, 'Whatever is nourished grows and flourishes, whatever is neglected and left unnourished decays and dies'.

The restraints of Yama and the practices of Niyama are not the morals and ethics which vary from culture to culture. They are not limited by social or political circumstances nor by any geographical or temporal factors. Yama and Niyama are discovered through practice, not through discussion, to be universal truths which require no apologetic justifications. They are the foundations of yoga practice.

Not everyone will achieve all the skills and have all the experiences which are required to enable them to transcend vitarka. To speed progress certain physical and mental exercises are useful. Perhaps the greatest initial problem for most people is their inability to be still. Few people are able to sit still for more than a little while without practice, and it is even rarer to be able to still the mind without training. Yoga is the science of stillness. As when starting a race, an athlete adopts a suitable posture which will ensure the best possible start, so in yoga there are postures which may be adopted to speed progress. These are the *Asanas*—the third stage of yoga experience. They have a very large mental component which is not always obvious to the onlooker but is the vital element which helps the practitioner gain physical and mental stability.

Having overcome the major difficulties in starting to clear the personality of confusion, the next stage is one of expansion. *Prana* means 'energy' and *ayama* means 'expansion'. The fourth stage of yoga—*Pranayama*—is one of expanding our awareness beyond its initial limited and restricted horizons. It is scientifically as well as spiritually true to say that everything we experience is ourself. It has been suggested that our mind is the produce of our brain states and even that our mental experience is our brain processes. At the same time, today we have experimental evidence which clearly shows that all our experience is not of the external world immediately, but is mediated. Even the most materialistic scientist must admit that we do not experience the universe as it really is. Rather we experience our own response to the universe. All our experience is experience of ourself. There is no doubt that we can experience our brain. It may be seen, touched, smelled or even tasted. The brain is undoubtedly a construction of our own mental experience. It is hypothetical that our mental experience is the product of our brain. If we state that our mental experience is the product of our mental experience, which is what an elaborated argument might boil down to, we have created a circular argument, a tautology. However, one of the statements is dubious and the other is *a priori*. Something has got to give and we are left with the proper conclusion that our brain is the product of our mind. The idea that the mind is the product of the brain is pure wishful thinking by those who are not prepared to face up to the real challenge of life. It is not seriously supported by any experimental evidence.

Nevertheless, we tend to identify with our physical brains and bodies and mentally create a dividing line between our bodies and the environment. This demarcation of personal identity is completely arbitrary. We have power over everything with which we identify completely. Within our bodies we are hardly aware of any organ or tissue, much less have any measure of control over it, but when we are fully aware of our heart, for example, we may slow down its beating and stop it at will without any physical ill-effects. This has been demonstrated by yogis under exacting scientific conditions.[1] Through expanding our awareness we may gain greater and greater power over ourselves as body and environment. Through practice of Pranayama we may expand beyond our ego image. Instead of remaining imprisoned in our body image we may discover experientially what physics already knows—that we are omnipresent beings. Through Pranayama we regain entrance to the wonderful realms of the universe that we

25

have denied ourselves for so long. It is a process of transforming our individual energy into cosmic energy.

Having come alive to the world we live in, we are then ready to come alive to the world that lives within ourselves. Having expanded our consciousness in a horizontal direction, we may also extend it in a vertical direction. The fifth step—*Pratyhara*—entails a collecting together of our dispersed psychic energies for the purpose of discovering greater depths of reality.

Sometimes yoga practice is divided into two aspects, Hatha and Raja. Hatha Yoga is considered to be concerned primarily with the stages of yoga experience so far discussed, which are external, and Raja Yoga is considered to be more concerned with the following stages, which are internal. To practise Hatha Yoga without Raja Yoga is considered useless by most traditional teachers, such as Swami Svatmarama who wrote the classic text *Hathapradipika*[2]. To practise Hatha Yoga is like preparing for a trip but never actually going on it. Again, few people are able to practise Raja Yoga unless they rid themselves of the inhibitions that would prevent them from making any real progress: this, Hatha Yoga is designed to do. The purpose of Hatha Yoga is to prepare the personality by stilling the habitual activity of body and mind to produce a clarity through which the light of Self may shine.

The sixth step of yoga is called *Dharana*. *Dhara* indicates a 'flow' and refers to the experience of thoughts and ideas which continuously flow through our minds. The great difficulty is to transcend these mental disturbances, and the problem is tackled by fixing the mind on certain points, internal and external.

Dhyana, the seventh step of yoga, is in some ways an extension of the attention exercises of the previous stage. Continuous attention is concentration. *Dhyana* means 'entering into', and through meditation we may pass beyond the appearance of the world and enter into a deeper understanding of life. At this point in our psychological development we realise that the universe that we experience is the result of suggestion. Through practice of Dhyana we may suggest all the qualities which we wish to manifest, removing, through meditation, all the old suggestions that have previously limited our lives. Suggestions like 'I am not intelligent enough . . . ', 'I am not able to . . . ' and countless others, are responsible for our major experience of limitation. Through positive suggestion we may achieve almost anything. Once it was thought impossible that man could go to the moon, but he has achieved it through the power of the imagination. These space trips are as nothing compared with the cosmic trips which are available through practice of Dhyana.

The eighth stage of yoga is *Samadhi*—an absolute state of identification. Dharana maintained for some while becomes Dhyana, and Dhyana sustained over a length of time becomes Samadhi. *Sam* means 'complete and absolute', and Samadhi is a complete state of concentration. Through our power to concentrate we learn quickly. Learning is self-discovery, as nothing is experienced but ourself scientifically. It is the process of transforming non-self into Self. Through Samadhi it is possible for us to expand our consciousness from individuality to universality, and in doing this we may realise that all is Self.

When consciousness is totally expanded through direct experience of the universe as Self, a state known as Samadhi Saguna is achieved. When no separation is experienced at all and the universe no longer exists, then that is the state of Samadhi Nirguna (see Chapter 16). This is the end point towards which all evolution is directed. It has great reality but no dimension.

3 Yama and Niyama— The Entrance Qualifications for Yoga

There are very real and definite entrance qualifications for yoga. They are the yamas and niyamas, which consist of things which should be taken in hand and restrained, and things which should be reinforced and practised. No one can make any real progress in self-discovery until they master Yama and Niyama, for they deal with the fundamental things which tend to cloud the mirror of personality which reflects the Self.

Traditionally there are five classes of Yama and five classes of Niyama.

Yama

The first yama is called *Ahimsa. Himsa* means 'killing, violence, or injury' and with the 'a' prefix it means 'non-violence'.

There are three main manifestations of violence, the first, most obviously, being physical violence. The history of the world is very much the history of war. Practically every culture has moved through periods of great violence and war, followed by periods of greater tranquillity. But men soon forget the horrors of war and continually resort to physical violence to effect changes in the world; and as that which is wrought by the sword can only be maintained by the sword, the periodic cycles of violence necessarily continue.

Superiority is often associated with physical dominance, which tends to encourage the practice of violent sports and competitions under the guise of cultural activity. We live in a world of muggings and senseless maiming, but newspapers, magazines, television and cinema all capitalise on violence to such an extent that our minds are often dulled to what it really is. Countless modern heros, such as James Bond, glorify violence.

Violence can also be manifested verbally. We talk of the cold war and psychological warfare. The vocal violence of one politician depreciating another is cheered on by keen supporters. The spiteful word, the sarcastic comment, the acid humour, are all examples of verbal violence. The suggestions that another should 'drop dead', 'get stuffed' and so on are frequently overheard, even in friendly conversation.

It is fairly easy to refrain from physical violence in a highly inhibited society where the law says that you will be punished if you do not; it is not so very difficult to refrain from verbal violence; but mental violence runs riot everywhere. There are the simple examples of mentally wishing a person ill, but there are also subtler instances; for example, many people do their own bodies and minds great violence by taking narcotics. You can kill ideals and innocence as easily as annihilating a fly in summer. Even tolerance of violence is against Ahimsa. Only by cultivating positive non-violent thoughts, and by banishing violent acts and speech, can Ahimsa be established. If an individual has fully achieved Ahimsa all living beings will cease their aggression in his presence.

The second yama is *Satyama*, which means 'truthfulness'. This does not involve merely the absence of falsehood and lies. It includes this but goes far beyond it. Many people find truthfulness a very difficult requirement. We live in a society that condones the absence of truth, accepting that its leaders, such as politicians and scientists, do not always tell the truth. Propaganda and advertising invariably rely on partial truth and, in some instances, pure lies or manipulated statistics. The question 'What is truth?' is asked only by those who do not lead truthful lives, for the meaning of truth is self-evident to all who live by the light of truth. Those who live a life of lies are confused and cannot perceive truth, even when faced with it themselves. The confidence trickster may ultimately deny himself life by believing it to be just another con.

Complete trust is impossible in a world of lies. Many relationships at personal, national and international level break down through lack of trust. A yogi neither trusts nor distrusts but checks his facts and perceives things as they are. He is neither gullible nor cynical, but accepts the universe as it is. His world is built on the solid rock of verifiable truth, not on the shifting sands of opinion and false assumption. The yogi is thus a realist while the non-yogi is an escapist, seeking to avoid the truth of the universe.

Truth, however, should not be used for the purposes of destruction. To use it in such a manner is but a simulation of virtue. Truth should be spoken for the benefit of all beings. First of all it is vital to be truthful with yourself, for self-deception about your own behaviour and attainments is only too easy. When your mind is completely truthful all your actions will bear positive fruit immediately. When a man lives and entertains the truth alone he becomes a source of enlightenment to all others.

The third class of yama is *Asteya* which means 'non-stealing'. There are many levels on which we can steal, be it a free bus ride or stealing a book from a library. While very few people in the West would actually carry out a robbery, considerably more people are prepared to accept stolen property or steal on the pretext that they have a right to take a certain amount from others who can afford it. Industry and particularly the wholesale and retail companies in the West allow a definite percentage of their turnover to vanish without trace, euphemistically calling this stealing 'shrinkage'. It would be difficult to estimate how much time is 'stolen' from employers by idling staff smoking in the lavatory or playing cards behind a wall of packing cases. 'Backhanders' and bribes given to public servants in decision-making positions by large construction firms have only recently been exposed in the newspapers. It is nothing new. In India it is almost impossible to do any business without bribery. It is a sign of the times that the sacred symbol *Aum* is painted on the backs of vehicles in India to indicate to the police that a certain bribe has been paid and that the vehicle and driver may be permitted to break the law of the land unmolested.

Ideas may also be stolen, and some people are adept at stealing the credit for work that others have done. It is the inner attitude which matters most for outward behaviour will follow. When you attain the state of Asteya you will have renounced all personal property. In giving up all possessions the whole universe becomes your property.

Brahmacharya is the fourth class of yama. It is the practice of devoting your life to the study of the highest aspects of Self. As has been said, it is scientifically true to say that everything we experience is ourself, and therefore the practice of seeing everything as Self is simply a matter of putting things into their correct perspective. However, most of us are fighting ourselves: we feel threatened and challenged by other egos; we are insecure and full of anxiety; we place ourselves in a disadvantageous position in life. Being internally divided we are easy prey for the negative suggestions which prowl around the universe hunting down the weakest. Predators are nature's agents for keeping a species healthy and thriving, and if the natural predators are removed the species deteriorates, becomes soft, diseased and dies out. The history of man has countless examples of societies which have removed all natural opposition and have then become lazy and decadent. The result has always been a decline and fall followed by a renaissance.

If you practise Brahmacharya and regard everything as Self, then you are indeed manifesting the golden rule that has been at the basis of every moral philosophy. By realising that all is Self and by applying that realisation you will become effectively selfless and will be truly unselfish. If, however, your previous conditioning will not allow you to face up to the scientific fact that all is Self, you will create and maintain a tension which is experienced as desire. An equal and opposite force will then be generated by the energies of separation which you are manifesting. This force is the energy of unification, known to all men as the sex drive—the fundamental spiritual drive to experience all as Self.

Once more, this drive may be expressed at many different levels. For example, it may be expressed at the physical level when it is interpreted as physical sexual desire. Sexuality, however is not simply a physical thing. The lowest and least satisfying expression of sexuality is the physical, yet most people place a great deal of importance in this aspect and base their lives on attaining fulfilment at this level. A lot of people are frustrated. They imagine sex, read about it, see films which feature it, plan it, talk about it and practise it, but get so involved with it that they can get no real satisfaction from it. Having invested so much conscious energy in sex, they have very little left to do anything of real value. Only when you can free your consciousness from this psycho-sexual tangle can you begin to make real progress in yoga.

However, merely repressing your psycho-sexual desires is of little use as you still have the problem but are simply not acknowledging it. There are of course many other ways of experiencing separation in the world but by far the most powerful block to progress in yoga is the sexual one, and for that reason

30

Brahmacharya is sometimes inadequately translated as 'continence'. This is misleading, for most of the ancient exponents of yoga were happily married men with families, and a fulfilled sex life in a proper context is not an obstacle to the practice of Brahmacharya. If a yogi is married to a woman who is a yogini in her own right, she is called yogipatni.

When you perfect the practice of Brahmacharya and experience the whole universe as Self, then you obtain incredible physical, psychological and spiritual strength.

The last yama is *Aparigraha—Graha* meaning approximately 'grab'. The accumulation of material wealth is a standard psychological drive. Amassing and hoarding possessions far in excess of what we really need is considered to be success in the world. There are many who think that the test of being clever is whether you are rich. In a more subtle way we are sometimes content to go without riches and worldly wealth in order to acquire worldly fame and recognition. We sell our integrity very cheaply, as politicians and other public figures will to get votes or publicity.

In order to be free to pursue the important things in life it is necessary to overcome the desire to hoard possessions or wealth for personal use. Aparigraha does not imply total rejection of material things, but requires that the yogi understands the real value and use of money and the effective use to which material things can be put to free man from some of the more mundane chores of life. Aparigraha is the practice of using tools and possessions properly without hoarding them unnecessarily.

Gandhi said 'There is enough for every man's need on earth, but not enough for every man's greed'. In order to grow in yoga, material possessions—psychological or physical—cannot be placed before everything else. If your possessions possess you, occupying your time and energy maintaining and protecting them, you will not be free to practise yoga. When you are able to live in this world without attachment to material things, you will have achieved Aparigraha. Through an understanding of attachment, achieved by mastering non-attachment, you will gain an insight into all your relationships and why you have been born in the body you are presently occupying.

Niyama

The first niyama is *Saucha*, which means 'purity'. In practising Hatha Yoga you will produce all kinds of endocrine and exocrine secretions, therefore, it is important to keep your body clean inwardly and outwardly. Every aspect of life is included in yoga practice, for your clothes, just as much as your actions are a description of your personality and so is your immediate environment. Pollution is as much a psychological problem as a social or environmental one.

The practice of cleanliness starts with your body, proceeds to your clothes and your rooms, and expands into everything. Do you carelessly throw your litter away at a picnic or on a bus rather than dispose of it properly? A lot of people are concerned only with appearances, wearing dirty underwear beneath their fineries or sweeping the dust underneath the carpet at home. You have only to see a football stadium after a match to see the incredible mess which is a collective description of the crowd.

Then there is purity of speech. Whilst some things may be enough to make a saint swear, the yogi must resist and manifest only beauty in his speech. Foul language does not usually lead to enlightenment, but can often lead to ugly situations which are unnecessary. It has been said that it does not matter what goes in to the mouth of a man, what comes out is the important thing. Speech is the major means of communication, and as the yogi is concerned with establishing a positive, unpolluted community which will be conducive to yoga practice, he observes Saucha.

Perhaps mental purity is the most difficult to attain, but by constant concentration of pure thoughts the mind can be cleared for effective higher work. If the mirror of the mind is muddied it cannot reflect the Self clearly and enlightenment is impossible. Through practice of Saucha you will obtain an immunity from the physical and psychological pollution around you, and having cleared your mind you will become serene and be in a position to perceive directly the nature of Self.

The second niyama is *Santosha*, which means 'contentment'. Through lack of contentment we are unable to enjoy even the present and we miss the beauty of life around us by always looking to the future or to the past, searching for a greener hill, overlooking the lush pasture on which we are standing. Santosha is not lack of ambition—the yogi is ultimately ambitious for his aim is to realise the highest goal—but the yogi is in harmony with the world and does not argue with it. He experiences the present as being good, proper and correct, providing him with all he needs in life. This contentment brings great happiness and when you are happy work is easy and your life is fulfilled.

Tapasya, the third niyama, is the practice of self-discipline (tapa). Discipline is the condition in which maximum learning can take place, and tapa entails proper use of your senses to maximise your yogic progress. Variations in temperature and environment, pleasures and pains, comforts and discomforts must all be overcome in order to guarantee maximum learning at all times. Do not confuse yourself by thinking about life and what you are doing, but at the same time be aware, observe and be attentive in all things you do. Through Tapasya, your life will become concentrated and you will soon perfect your body, mind and senses.

The fourth niyama is *Svadhiyaya*, the study of physics, metaphysics and all the human sciences with the aim of understanding the organisation of the universe which is Self. The yogi is a scientist who studies all the branches not only of modern but also of ancient science. His study is directed and meaningful, not simply the accumulation of useless information. *Svadhiyaya* means 'study' or 'application', and through applying your mind to the study of everything in the universe you will discover and communicate with the whole of nature and the truth that all is Self will be actualised and manifested.

The fifth niyama is called *Ishvarapranidhanani*. *Vara* means 'vibration' and *Ishvara* 'the totality of vibration', ie the universe of energy and matter. *Pranidhanani* is the process of identification and hence the fifth niyama—Ishvarapranidhanani—is the practice of identifying with the entire universe of vibration so that the limited ego may become cosmic. Just as you attain body consciousness by identifying with your body, so you will undoubtedly attain cosmic consciousness by identifying with the entire cosmos.

4 The Chakra System 1

Much of Hatha Yoga practice is designed to free our communication blocks to awaken the chakras. The practical techniques which are described in this book require a knowledge of the chakra system, which is the key to all scientific knowledge. It is the summation of ancient scientific discoveries and is destined to be recognized once more as the model upon which all complete systems are based. Modern science is about to catch up with ancient yoga science and it will be the greatest scientific break-through of our present era.

Yoga is based on science of a very high level. About two thousand years ago, Patanjali, one of the greatest systemizers of yoga, wrote an extremely authoritative work beginning 'Atha yoganushasanam. . . '. Dr. Mishra, perhaps the most qualified translator of this text alive today, interprets Patanjali as follows: 'The term atha indicates that a distinct topic begins here. It means that after completing study of all branches of physics and metaphysics, yoga should be practised'.[1]

This is a daunting requirement, but only after considerable scientific education is it possible to fully appreciate yoga literature and practice. In yoga literature it is said 'How can there be any attainment (siddhi) for him who does not know the six chakras, the sixteen adharas, the five pranas and the three lingas in his own body'?

Unfortunately it is not within the scope of this work to give more than a brief introduction to the chakras. This chapter and the next two are designed to give you a feel for the biological basis of yoga practice. Readers with an interest in the scientific foundation of yoga may wish to refer to our book *Both Sides of the Brain*.

The Traditional Chakra System

The manifest universe is a universe of vibrating energy, Prana. It is a universe of music, and its laws are those of music. If we can truly understand any one octave of vibration then we have an insight into every octave in the universe because each one is in resonance with all other octaves of energy everywhere.

We may experience the octave aurally as the seven notes on a piano scale, or we may experience it visually as the spectrum of colour. The structure of the atom, with its seven electronic shells, is based on the

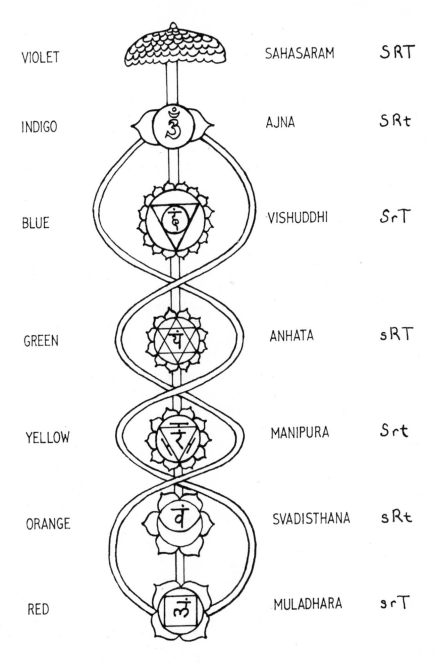

VIOLET		SAHASARAM	S R T
INDIGO		AJNA	S R t
BLUE		VISHUDDHI	S r T
GREEN		ANHATA	s R T
YELLOW		MANIPURA	S r t
ORANGE		SVADISTHANA	s R t
RED		MULADHARA	s r T

The traditional chakra system

octave, and the solar system is constructed on a harmonic plan. At every level of existence energies manifest the form of the octave. From macro-cosm to microcosm the pattern known as the chakra system is evident. Echoing this truth the Vishvasara Tantra says:

What is here is elsewhere
What is not here is nowhere.

The traditional chakra[2] system seen in yogic texts is a mnemonic aid designed to summarise the important features of the pattern. There is a central path called the Sushumna. Six centres are spaced at intervals along this meridian and a seventh somewhat larger centre is at the top. A chakra is a centre and may be thought of as a nodal point. Starting in the lowest centre and terminating in the sixth are two curved paths known as the Ida and Pingala.

According to yoga theory everything in the universe is composed of three qualities (gunas) which are never found separately yet manifest in every possible combination. Different states of matter, physical, biological or psychological are distinguished by their relative proportions of the three gunas; sattoguna (S), rajoguna (R) and tamoguna (T). In one model of the chakra system each chakra may be associated with its guna combination by denoting a dominant component with S,R,T and a recessive component by s,r,t. This leads to a seven level model (ignoring the combination 'srt' as it is essentially a similar balance to 'SRT' although at a lower resonance).

The chakra system is the archetypal form of the universe. The personological manifestation of the system is described in the first chapter, but for our purposes it is useful to see this pattern reflected in the life processes manifested in a biological cell.

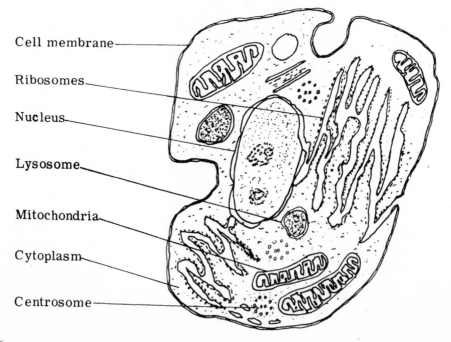

Cell membrane

Ribosomes

Nucleus

Lysosome

Mitochondria

Cytoplasm

Centrosome

The cells which make up the human body have all descended from a single fertilised ovum. This one cell has divided and subdivided according to the millions of years of memory which it stores in the DNA molecules contained in its tiny nucleus. Every new cell contains exactly the same memories yet each new cell takes on some specialist role. Groups of similar cells compose tissues which are arranged to form organs and these organs are themselves grouped into systems which all work together as a whole. These systems also reflect the pattern of the chakra system. The health of the body and its integral functioning depends upon the successful co-ordination and communication of every member.

The body (annamayakosh) is made of food (anna) which is borrowed from the environment for a while and returned. Before birth our mother provides the substances which energize and build our physical being. Afterwards we

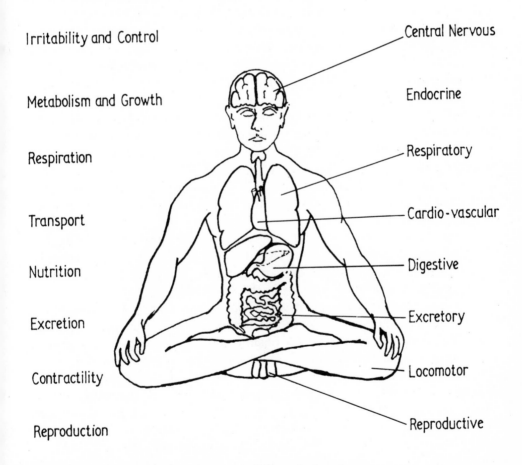

Irritability and Control

Metabolism and Growth

Respiration

Transport

Nutrition

Excretion

Contractility

Reproduction

Central Nervous

Endocrine

Respiratory

Cardio-vascular

Digestive

Excretory

Locomotor

Reproductive

The essential life processes as delegated to the different body systems absorb the necessary material through our intestine and lungs. During the growth phase we excrete less material than we take in but the turn-over of body constituents continues all our life. The body as a whole may survive eighty years but its cells, from brain to bone, will have been replaced many times. Their chemical constituents are turned over even more rapidly. This constant change is called metabolism. Its constructive phase is anabolism (kapha) and its destructive phase, catabolism (pitta). The management and maintenance of these processes (vatta) is carried out by modulating the ion fluxes and cyclic AMP levels of the individual cells through cell membrane mediated communication. This has reached evolutionary specialization in neural transmission and hormone action, respectively.

The developing embryo takes on a form which depends on the electromagnetic life-field it grows in and retains until death. Three major tissues arise; the ectoderm, mesoderm and endoderm. They are relatively, sattvic, rajsic and tamsic in quality, respectively. Skeletal muscle forms from the mesoderm and the viscera develops from endoderm. The tissue which has folded in on its self to form a tube. The inside of the tube is the cerebrospinal canal and is extremely sensitive to a wide range of electromagnetic, chemical and other stimuli. The outside of the tube is the much less sensitive but all-important skin. The inner part of the tube thickens to produce the central nervous system (CNS) called the *sushumna* in Sanskrit. It is composed of the brain and spinal cord which lie entirely within the vertebral column and the skull. It retains its connections to the skin through the sensory part of the peripheral nervous system (PNS) (*parisarya nadi mandalam* in Sanskrit) which enters the CNS from the back. Communication with most of the rest of the body is achieved through the autonomic nervous system (ANS).

The nervous system is largely composed of perineural cells called glia in the CNS and Schwann in the PNS. These cells form a continuous DC electrical network connected by gap junctions. They are the earliest and most fundamental control system in the body. At the central areas of the CNS they are electrically positive becoming more and more negative in polarity as they move towards the periphery and down the arms and legs. This DC system is responsible for healing and repair functions in the body. It conducts primary body feelings and pain information to the CNS. It is an analog system which is sensitive to environmental electromagnetic (EM) changes. It conditions the immediate environment for the evolutionarily more recent digital communication system provided by nerve cells (neurons). Most nerve cells maintain a certain independence from each other and communicate via chemical messengers such as GABA, Dopamine, Epinephrine and Acetylcholine, which are known as neurotransmitters. Very complicated arrangements of nerve cells have evolved and intricate chemical processes determine whether the ionic state of a neuron will be disturbed or not. If it is, then a fast AC message may be relayed along its length to release chemicals from its terminal points which may stimulate or inhibit other neurons or effector organs such as the muscles and internal organs.

The spinal column (meru danda) houses the spinal cord and is divided into five sections: the coccyx, the sacral, lumbar, thoracic and cervical regions. These represent the Muladhara, Svadisthana, Manipura, Anahata and Vishuddhi Chakras respectively. The general cross section of the spinal cord shows a grey H-shaped portion (chitra nadi) which consists of local nerve networks. This is surrounded by a white area (vajra nadi) which is composed of vertical nerve tracts carrying messages to and from higher and lower levels. In the center of the 'H' is a small hole which is the continuation of the cerebrospinal canal and is known as the brahmanadi in yoga. The spinal cord (sushumna kandam) is about 17 inches long and reaches from the second lumbar vertebra to the base of the skull where it is continuous with the brain stem. Thirty one pairs of nerves emerge from the spinal cord: eight cervical nerves supply the muscles of the neck, arms and the hands; twelve thoracic nerves supply the trunk and intercostal muscles; the five lumbar and the upper sacral nerves supply the legs and feet; the lower sacral nerves supply the anal and perineal muscles. Nerves regulating the muscular system are associated with *udana*.

The Autonomic Nervous System

The ANS may be divided into the sympathetic division, with nerves leaving the spinal cord from the thoracic and lumbar segments, and the parasympathetic division, with nerves leaving from the cranial and sacral segments. (See diagram.)

The sympathetic division represents the Pingala and is associated with the right nostril (surya) in Pranayama. It tends to act in a widespread manner to prepare the body for emergencies and vigorous musclar activity. When the sympathetic system is activated there is an increase of cardiovascular and respiratory activity; gastro-intestinal activity is curtailed, glucose is released from glycogen stores, blood in channelled to the muscles and excess heat is removed by sweating. The pupils of the eyes dilate, the eyes tend to protrude and the eyelids widen. This general activity is known as adrenergic.

In addition to this massive activity during emergencies, the various parts of the sympathetic division function in everyday life in independent and discrete ways. Fine control of the ANS may be learned through yoga practices.[3]

The parasympathetic division is known as the Ida in yoga and is associated with the left notstril (chandra). The parasympathetic division acts more discretely on individual organs or regions. The abdominal viscera are innervated by neurons which leave the cranial part of the cord and travel via the vagus nerves. The branches of the vagus consist mainly of sensory afferents which participate in the samana activity as visceral reflexes, such as those of the abdomen and the pressure and chemical receptors in the aortic arch and the heart. The sacral part of the parasympathetic division is primarily concerned with apana functions such as the emptying of the pelvic organs and with reproductive functions.

Whereas the sympathetic division is mainly involved with homeostasis during voluntary activity, the parasympathetic division is involved with restorative vegetative functions such as digestion and rest. Parasympathetic activity is generally known as cholinergic. Briefly, sympathetic dominance is associated with a more active, rajsic state and parasympathetic dominance with a more receptive, tamsic state.

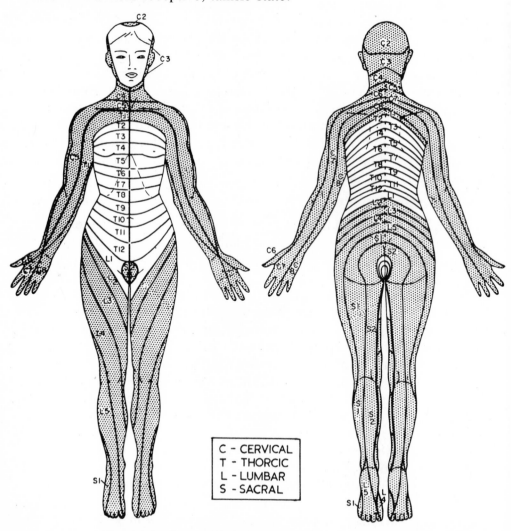

C – CERVICAL
T – THORCIC
L – LUMBAR
S – SACRAL

Diagram showing the skin innervated by nerves originating in the cervical, thoracic, lumbar and sacral regions of the spine

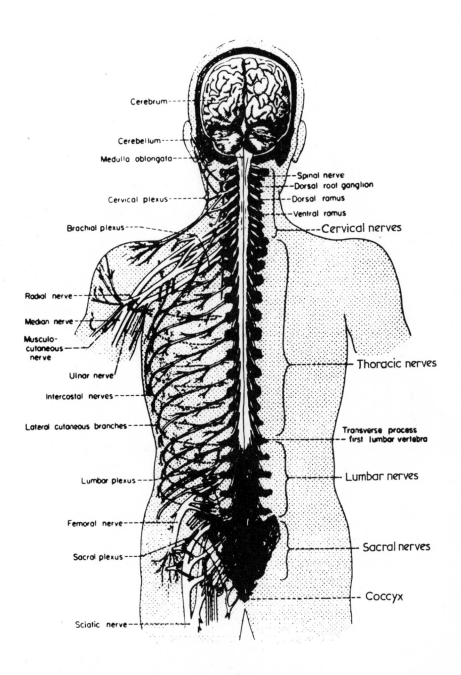

The nervous system in situ

41

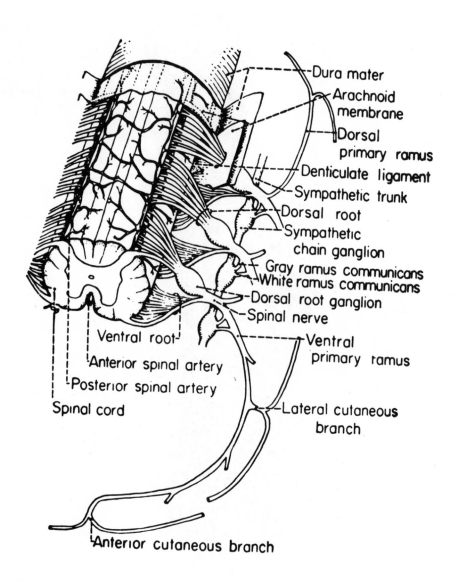

- Dura mater
- Arachnoid membrane
- Dorsal primary ramus
- Denticulate ligament
- Sympathetic trunk
- Dorsal root
- Sympathetic chain ganglion
- Gray ramus communicans
- White ramus communicans
- Dorsal root ganglion
- Spinal nerve
- Ventral primary ramus
- Lateral cutaneous branch

Ventral root
Anterior spinal artery
Posterior spinal artery
Spinal cord

Anterior cutaneous branch

The spinal cord in cross-section

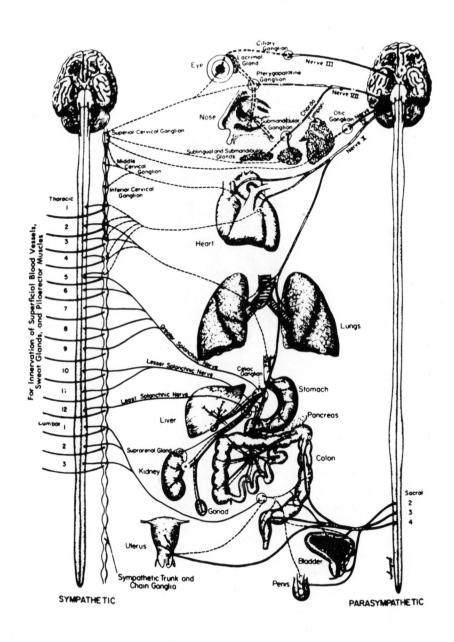

Plan of the autonomic system showing the
sympathetic and parasympathetic divisions

43

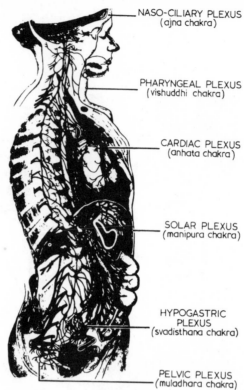

NASO-CILIARY PLEXUS
(ajna chakra)

PHARYNGEAL PLEXUS
(vishuddhi chakra)

CARDIAC PLEXUS
(anhata chakra)

SOLAR PLEXUS
(manipura chakra)

HYPOGASTRIC
PLEXUS
(svadisthana chakra)

PELVIC PLEXUS
(muladhara chakra)

The autonomic ganglia and plexuses

The brain

The top of the spinal cord enters the cranium and expands a little to become the medulla oblongata (meaning 'oblong marrow') and the pons (meaning 'bridge'). These structures are concerned with the biological functions of Prana and include centres for heart control, respiration and digestion. Here many of the verticle pathways of the CNS cross over from left to right and vice versa.

The central nervous system is basically a tube, and this tube expands to form a number of caverns, called the ventricles, at the centre of the brain. In yoga, the ventricles are of very great importance. The ascending cerebro-spinal canal, as the hole in the spinal cord is called, expands into the fourth ventricle between the pons and the cerebellum. This cavern is called the *shankini* in Sanskrit, which means 'the energy of the conch'. The fourth ventricle might be thought to look a little conch-shaped but the ancient rishis did not name the parts of the anatomy after their appearance, as they tended to do in the West thousands of years later. Rather they named them after their function. The conch sounds forth a great 'aum' sound when it is blown called the nada current. The word nada comes from a root word meaning 'motion'. The cerebellum (siro balam) is largely concerned with

44

motion and balance in the body while the pons acts as a bridge, connecting the lefthand functions with the right, and exerts influence on the auditory pathways.

The reticular formation is a net-like series of short, interwoven fibres and nerve cells about the size of your little finger. It extends from the medulla, through the pons and the midbrain, up into the thalamus. The reticular formation underlies our awareness of the world and our ability to think and act. It plays the role of a sentinel which arouses the cortex and has been called the reticular activating system (RAS). The RAS exercises some control over reflex reactions and can also enhance or inhibit information going towards the brain, or processes taking place in the spinal column, rather like a traffic control centre.

When the brain is alert, conscious and is fully manifesting, and when the energies of action and motion in the body are in equilibrium, then the individual hears a sound rather like that of the conch. The sound is not localised in the ears but seems to come from everywhere. This is the nada current. Yogis hear the nada sound all the time but to a varying extent according to the level of yogic attainment and the degree of consciousness manifested.

The sound 'aum' is sometimes called the pranava. Here 'pranava' indicates the entry of Prana into the body through the medulla oblongata which borders the fourth ventricle. The respiratory centres are controlled through the effects of hydrogen ions in the cerebrospinal fluid filling the fourth ventricle. Prana enters into the body in a number of ways but its most important entrance is through the medulla oblongata via the fourth ventricle during deep sleep.

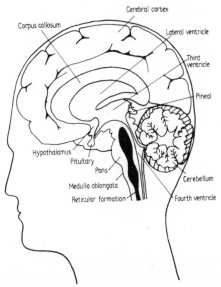

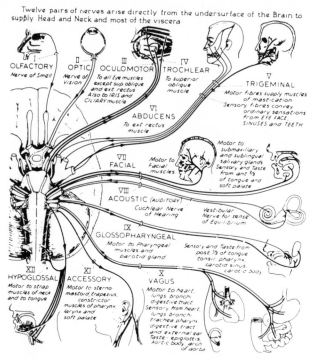

Twelve pairs of nerves arise directly from the undersurface of the Brain to supply Head and Neck and most of the viscera

I OLFACTORY Nerve of Smell

II OPTIC Nerve of Vision

III OCULOMOTOR To all eye muscles except sup.oblique and ext.rectus Also to IRIS and CILIARY muscle

IV TROCHLEAR To superior oblique muscle

V TRIGEMINAL Motor fibres supply muscles of mastication Sensory fibres convey ordinary sensations from EYE FACE, SINUSES and TEETH

VI ABDUCENS To ext.rectus muscle

VII FACIAL Motor to Facial muscles Motor to submaxillary and sublingual salivary glands Sensory and Taste from ant. ⅔ of tongue and soft palate

VIII ACOUSTIC (AUDITORY) Cochlear Nerve of Hearing Vestibular Nerve for sense of Equilibrium

IX GLOSSOPHARYNGEAL Motor to Pharyngeal muscles and parotid gland Sensory and Taste from post.⅓ of tongue tonsil pharynx, carotid sinus, carotid body

XII HYPOGLOSSAL Motor to strap muscles of neck and to tongue

XI ACCESSORY Motor to sterno mastoid, trapezius, constrictor muscles of pharynx, larynx and soft palate

X VAGUS Motor to heart, lungs bronchi, digestive tract Sensory from heart, lungs bronchi, trachea pharynx digestive tract and external ear Taste - epiglottis, Aortic body, arch of aorta

The cranial nerves and their function

The hypothalamus

The hypothalamus and lower brain centres represents the Ajna chakra. It is the head ganglia of the ANS and the centre which interrelates the visceral and somatic functions of the body. It is situated below the thalamus which may be considered as a relay centre connecting the hypothalamus with other brain centres. In yoga literature it is called the triveni, which means 'the place where the three rivers meet', because the Ida, Pingala and Sushumna meet at this point.

It is interesting to note that not only are motor actions accompanied by widespread and complex visceral responses, but visceral activity modifies somatic reactions. For instance, during digestion the increased blood flow through the intestines tends to reduce the musclar capacity for work. The hypothalamus is associated with vyana and concerns regulations of:

1 The cardiovascular system

2 Respiration

3 Body temperature

4 Body water and electrolyte concentrations

5 Food intake and gastric pancreatic secretions

46

6   Pituitary secretion, sexual and maternal behaviour

7   Emotional states

In yoga science we know that the hypothalamus is programmed by neural impulses coming from the olfactory lobes and nasal sinuses which may be consciously controlled through yoga training.

The cerebral aquaduct is a narrow tube that connects the fourth ventricle to the third ventricle above it. The third ventricle is called sunyadesha in yoga and is perhaps the most important place in the body. *Sunya* means 'radiant ether'; *desha* means 'origin' or 'the natural source'. The sunyadesha is in the very centre of the head. Here the plasmic structure of the cerebrospinal fluid is modulated by the earth's electromagnetic changes which in turn is affected by activity of the ionosphere, which is influenced by solar and cosmic events.

Two parallel caverns lead off from the third ventricle and these are the lateral ventricles which occupy the centres of the right and left cerebral hemispheres. They are crescent-shaped and are lined, like the third and fourth ventricles, with the choroid plexus. The choroid plexus is called the *chandra* in Sanskrit which means the 'moon'. As the moon is associated with water and tides so the choroid plexus is associated with fluids, producing cerebrospinal fluid (CSF) from blood. There is a general slow movement of CSF through the ventricles and down into the cerebrospinal canal where it is absorbed back in into the venous system. The cerebrospinal canal system only contains about 150ml of CSF, the fluid is replaced six or seven times each day. This fluid is called *amrit* in Sanskrit, which means 'life giving'. It deserves this name as it directs all our life functions through its effects on the CNS.

The cerebral cortex

We have two brains which together form the cerebrum and represent the Sahasarum. It has the same name in Sanskrit, *sirobrahman,* which means 'the seat of consciousness'. The two brains appear superficially to be mirror images of each other, joined together by a large bundle of nerves called the corpus callosum. Each of the cerebral hemispheres is divided into four lobes: The frontal lobe; the parietal lobe, which is towards the top of the head; the occipital lobe, which is at the back of the head, and the temporal lobe, which is on the side beneath the temples. The outside of the cortex is grey matter and the inside is white matter—the reverse of the situation in the spinal cord.

Each hemisphere shares the potential for many functions and both sides participate in most activities. In the normal person, however, the two hemispheres tend to specialise. The left hemisphere is predominently involved with analytic, logical thinking, especially in verbal and mathematical functions. Its mode of operation is primarily linear and seems to process information sequentially. The right hemisphere seems to specialise in far

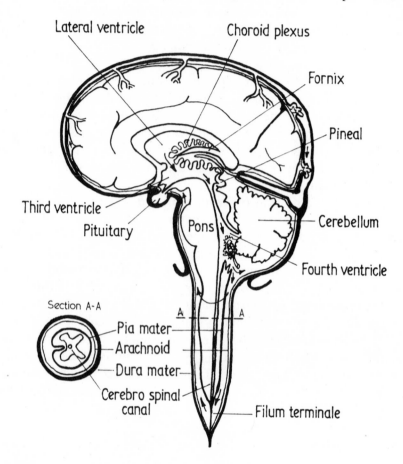

Lateral ventricle

Choroid plexus

Fornix

Pineal

Third ventricle

Pituitary

Pons

Cerebellum

Fourth ventricle

Section A-A

Pia mater
Arachnoid
Dura mater
Cerebro spinal canal

Filum terminale

more sensitive, receptive and holistic experience. This side is primarily responsible for our orientation in space, artistic endeavour, crafts, body image and recognition of faces.

This left/right differentiation has been standard knowledge in yoga from its beginnings, although it is just being discovered by the modern rishis of science. The left/right dichotomy is represented in yoga by the sun, surya, and the moon, chandra (not to be confused with the chandra as the choroid plexus). The sun makes an excellent symbol for the out-going, extroverted, active consciousness of the left brain, which finds its cultural expression predominantly in the West today. The moon perfectly symbolises the reflective, mystical, receptive consciousness of the right hemisphere, which finds its cultural expression in the East. In yoga these two complementary expressions of consciousness are represented by 'Ha' and 'Tha' and hence the name "Hatha' for the yoga practice which harmonises and synthesises these two aspects of personality.

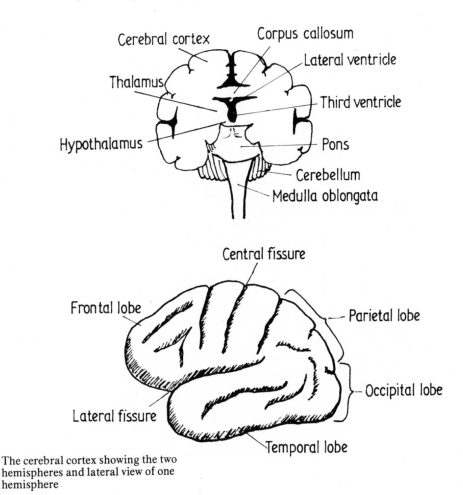

Cerebral cortex
Corpus callosum
Lateral ventricle
Thalamus
Third ventricle
Hypothalamus
Pons
Cerebellum
Medulla oblongata

Central fissure
Frontal lobe
Parietal lobe
Occipital lobe
Lateral fissure
Temporal lobe

The cerebral cortex showing the two hemispheres and lateral view of one hemisphere

Brain waves

In the widest possible sense it is true to say that everything in the universe is in vibration and is composed of waves. At one end of the spectrum of wavelength are the pulses set up by the billion year rotation of a galaxy and at the other are the incredibly short wavelengths of cosmic rays. Somewhere around halfway between these extremes lie the periodic rhythms of the earths EM standing waves and brain nerve activity.

The brain cells tend to act in patterns which set up electrical charges that may be detected on the surface of the scalp by sensitive electrodes. Roughly speaking the less the degree of harmony in the personality, the more agitated the brain waves appear. The brain waves are normally picked up by a machine called an electroencephalograph (EEG). Changes in brain waves have been shown to correlate with changes in the earth's magnetic field.

The fastest kind of brain wave pattern is called a beta rhythm and is associated with the psychological experiences of anxiety, forced attention, schizophrenia and mania, and with a generally high level of activity and involvement. A slower brain wave pattern activity of between 8 and 13 cycles per second, is called an alpha rhythm. It is associated with a relaxed state of mind, inwardly directed attention or lack of attention, passivity and a low level of activity and involvement in general. Slower still is the theta rhythm which is generally between 4 and 7cps and is associated with dreaming, access to 'unconscious' material, creative inspiration, visions, moderately deep meditation and receptivity to ESP. The slowest brain wave pattern of all is known as delta and consists of waves of less than about 4cps. Delta rhythm is associated with deep sleep, lack of perceptual awareness and very deep states of meditation.

The brain waves emanating from different parts of the brain may differ. For example, during verbal activity the alpha rhythm in the right hemisphere increases relative to the left while in a spatial activity the alpha increases in the left hemisphere relative to the right.

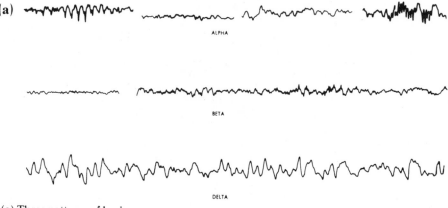

(a) Three patterns of brain wave

5 The Chakra System 11

The nervous system is concerned with the integration of the entire body through definite pathways and utilizes intricate information processing to relate internal and external events. In contrast the endocrine system modulates the internal environment through a much more generalized activity.

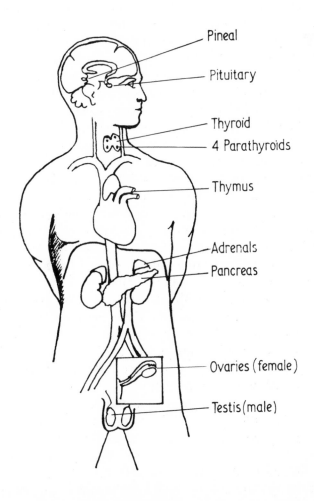

- Pineal
- Pituitary
- Thyroid
- 4 Parathyroids
- Thymus
- Adrenals
- Pancreas
- Ovaries (female)
- Testis (male)

The endocrine system

The Endocrine System

The endocrine system works in an analogous way to a broadcasting system. Hormones are secreted by certain glands directly into the bloodstream and circulate freely. Only specific body cells are 'tuned into' a particular hormone and pick up the chemical to respond to it. These cells are the 'target cells' for the hormone.

'Endocrine' comes from the Greek meaning to 'secrete within'. 'Hormone' is derived from a word meaning 'to excite or stimulate'. Several different hormones may be secreted from each endocrine gland and there are seven groups of these stimulating centres in the body. Many hormones are synthesized from single amino acids such as melatonin, thyroxine and epinephrine. Others are derived from chains of amino acids called polypeptides e.g., oxytocin, insulin, TSH. These hormones produce their effects by combining with specific receptors on the outside of the cell membrane rather like a key fits a lock. They do not enter the cell but unleash internal chemical processes when the enzyme adenyl cyclase is released to promote cyclic AMP synthesis which acts as a 'second messenger'.

Hormones act by regulating preexisting processes by influencing the rate of synthesis of enzymes and other proteins. They affect the rate of enzymatic catalysis and alter the permeability of cell membranes. A third group of hormones are steroids, derived from cholesterol e.g., estradiol, progesterone, cortisone. These are small molecules that actually enter into cells and are retained by target tissues when receptors in the cytoplasm combine with them and migrate to the genetic material in the nucleus. Specific genes are activated by each steroid hormone and this results in the synthesis of new proteins and other biological molecules.

The hormone producing centres are regulated by complicated feedback and feedforward processes. The biochemical pathways involved are both intriguing and of great practical relevance in yoga practice. Yogis have studied the behavioural and experiential correlates of the endocrine system for centuries using the general term 'ojas' for 'hormonal force'. Hormones do not just modulate our physiology but they determine the direction and quantity of a precise set of bodily processes. As most hormones are present in the blood plasma at any one time it is their relative quantities that determine the overall resultant of our psychosomatic state.

Every atom and molecule has its own unique set of energies and frequencies which may be observed by spectral analysis, nuclear magnetic resonance and other well established physical techniques. From quantom mechanical fluxation to galatic rotations everything dances to its own rhythm. Yet the rhythms of molecules, cells and solar systems are syncopated through gravitational, electromagnetic and other interactions.

The pineal

The endocrine equivalent of the sahasaram has been called the third eye. The pineal gland is a reddish, pine shaped organ about 0.4 in. long, which projects from the back of the third ventricle at the centre of our brain. It receives sympathetic stimulation by means of autonomic nerves which originate in the superior cervical ganglion of the neck. These connect with spinal tracts to the hypothalamus and the optic nerve. When our eyes detect light the information is shared with the pineal via this circuitous route. Earth interactions produce rhythms called the day, solar month, year etc., which are imposed on all biological entities as circadian rhythms (about a day), annual rhythms and so on. The pineal plays a principal role in conveying the geosolar rhythms to the rest of the body through its secretion of melatonin and other peptides. The daily sleep-waking cycle is associated with a 'sleep factor' which pours into the cerebrospinal fluid and effects the glial cells of the brain modifying the EEG and reversing the direct current potential between the back and front of the head.

Each night melatonin is produced and represses production of sex hormones providing a diurnal opportunity for higher creativity as the anti-gonadotrophic effect allows the imagination to transcend its psychosexual boundaries. A flush of gonadal hormones that comes around dawn tips the balance the other way inhibiting pineal activity. Melatonin has a very similsr structure to the hallucinogenic drugs psylocibin and LSD which may owe their mind-altering capabilities to their ability to mimic the natural hormone. Creative breakthroughs like babies, tend to arrive in the middle of the night.

The annual changes in length of daylight provide programming for sexual and physical activity. Heat production by the brown fat at the centre of our backs follows melatonins' waxing and waning. The winter Solstice, the darkest time of the year (in the Northern hemisphere) is traditionally a time for spiritual rebirth as new light and inspiration enters the inner world of humankind. Culturally it is celebrated in festivals such as Christmas and Hannukah.

Pineal tumours or other biochemical insufficiencies can overproduce melatonin and keep the possessor in the Peter Pan world of childlike fantasy and sexual unawareness. Pineal hypofunction in early life can lead to sexual precosity. Our imagination provides challenge and reveals possibility. When it malfunctions, our life looses purpose and we become depressed. Most pineals show signs of calcification at autopsy. Most of us begin the calcification and crystallization of our imagination at an early stage to provide a psychological prison which limits our whole life. Yoga is practised in the shade to avoid direct sunlight. Yoga is mastered when your imagination is liberated and becomes your most powerful creative tool inspiring the whole world. The image we hold governs our entire behaviour. The third eye enables us to see the world in a new light. The tuning of our pineal is revealed in the programme that is played out through our nervous system.

The pituitary

The endocrine equivalent of the ajna chakra is the pituitary. It protrudes from the base of the brain like a small mushroom and lies in its own special 'cave' in the floor of the cranium, called the Turkish saddle. The posterior pituitary is essentially an extension of the hypothalamus above. It is joined in fetal development by a piece of the primitive roof of the nasal cavity which forms the anterior pituitary. The join is called the pars intermedia and secretes melanocyte stimulating hormone (MSH) which may play a role in EM desensitization.

The anterior pituitary manufactures a number of peptide hormones in response to various releasing and inhibiting factors which are secreted into the circulation from cells in the hypothalamus. The pituitary has been called the 'master gland' because many of its anterior hormones stimulate the function of other endocrine glands. Thyrotrophin (TSH) stimulates the thyroid, Corticotrophin (ACTH) stimulates the cortex of the adrenals, and Gonadotrophins, (FSH,LH) stimulate different parts of the gonads. These organs secrete their products which find their way through the circulation to their target cells and to sites in the brain which complete a loop circuit. Higher brain centres modify the activity of the hypothalamus. Areas associated with emotional and intuitive experiences exert a major influence on pituitary function. Under psychological stress ACTH pours out to amplify corticosteroid production in the adrenals. This in turn depresses the immune system. The greater your psychological unease the more vulnerable you are to disease.

A particularly important hormone, Somatotrophin (G.H.) is secreted from the anterior pituitary. It acts with thyroxine and insulin to orchestrate complex metabolic processes. G.H. stands for 'growth hormone' which is its alternative name earned through its role in growth processes. Undersecretion in childhood produces a dwarf versus oversecretion which can produce giants of 7–8 feet. If it is overactive in an adult, the bones thicken, especially in the face, jaw, nose, hands and feet. There is a coarseness of the skin, and a condition called acromegaly results. Adult height is partly a result of child environmental ease. Yogis tend to have refined features.

The posterior pituitary secretes two interesting peptides. Vasopressin (ADH) conserves the body water by reducing water excretion by the kidneys, while oxytocin affects lactation and uterine muscle contraction. These hormones are synthesized in the hypothalamus and transported along nerves to the posterior pituitary where they are secreted into the circulation. Underactivity of ADH results in diabetes insipidus. Pituitary hormone production is very sensitive to the emotional state of the individual. Under intuitive insecurity or diffuse anxiety, symptoms such as infertility can arise. In the extreme case the entire output of the anterior pituitary can be so reduced that other endocrine organs begin to atrophy and the body

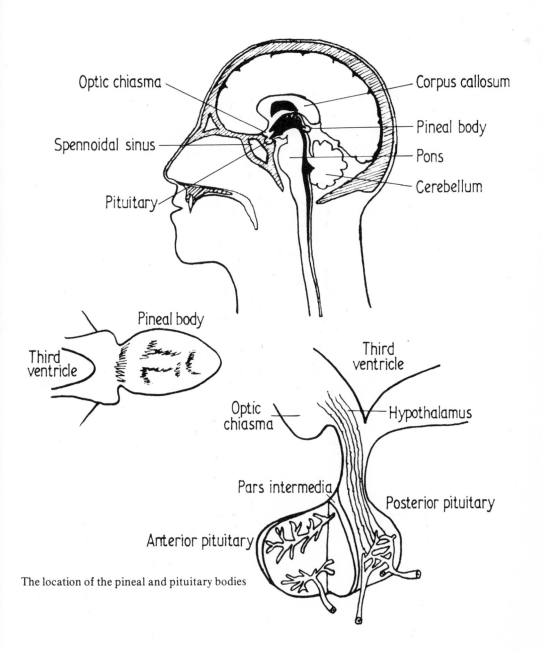

Optic chiasma

Corpus callosum

Pineal body

Pons

Spennoidal sinus

Cerebellum

Pituitary

Pineal body

Third ventricle

Third ventricle

Optic chiasma

Hypothalamus

Pars intermedia

Posterior pituitary

Anterior pituitary

The location of the pineal and pituitary bodies

becomes prematurely senile. In Sanskrit the pituitary is known as the *soma mandalam* and is associated with the moon through its role in mood and sexual cycles, growth and water control. The pituitary harmonizes the internal chemical environment to help relate the neurophysiological dilemma between its internal and external states. In response to the Vatt processes of the hypothalamus, kapha and pitta are modified.

The thyroid

The thyroid (meaning 'shield') is the endocrine equivalent of the Vishuddhi chakra. It is an H-shaped gland weighing about 25g, lying in front of the neck close to the larynx and trachea. Its principal hormone thyroxine affects oxygen consumption and heat production in the whole body by

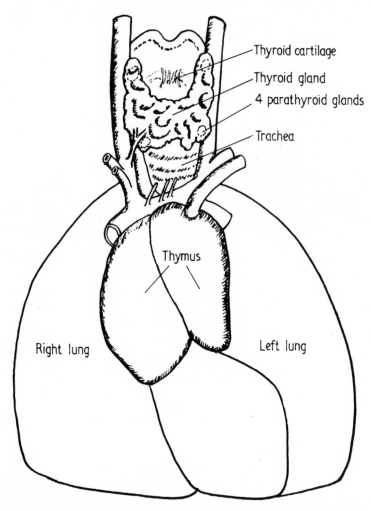

The thyroid, parathyroids and thymus glands

modulating the proticity in the respiratory systems of the mictochondria. Thyroxine (meaning 'to awaken') controls metabolic rate. Too much of the hormone produces a condition called hyperthyroidism characterised by a high amount of nervousness and emotionality, irritability, rapid reflexes and quick jerky movements. Typically such people have protruding eyeballs, although it is probably not due to this hormone. They burn up all the energy they have and so are usually skinny with a high colouring. Such a person feels warm even on cold days and is very uncomfortable in hot weather.

If the thyroid is underworking it produces a condition called hypothyroidism, characterised by a puffiness around the eyes, thick unshapely hands and a thickness around the base of the neck. The tongue becomes swollen and the voice rather hoarse. It is invariably a female condition. A person suffering from hypothyroidism is always cold and liabile to wear excessive clothing even in warm weather. She is very likely to gain weight, her pulse will be slow and alimentary tract lazy, resulting in constipation. Very often the hair begins to thin on top of the head. A lack of thyroid hormone in childhood results in cretinism. A cretin has a very low intelligence and a characteristically retarded appearance.

The simple goitre is a well known thyroid problem. It is the result of the thyroid growing considerably in size in an attempt to compensate for deficient hormone production. Insufficient thyroxin may be a result of lack of iodine and in some areas of the world where there is deficiency of iodine the goitre is endemic. In central China, for example, so many people have goitres that they are considered a thing of beauty. Some foods, such as Brussels sprouts, effectively destroy thyroid hormones, and if you were to eat such foods consistently and in large quantities you could develop a goitre.

A second major thyroid hormone, calcitonin, plays a complimentary role with parahormone which is produced in the parathyroids. These are four small brownish yellow pieces of tissue about the size and shape of flattened orange pits, applied to the back of the thyroid gland. Calcitonin and parahormone govern calcium homeostasis.

Under-production of parahormone is called hypoparathyroidism. In this condition calcium passes out of the blood into the tissues; the nerves become very excitable and muscle spasm—known as tetany—can occur or epileptic attacks may be provoked. Sometimes cataracts develop in the lenses of the eye, impairing vision. Calcification of parts of the brain, such as the pineal, can occur.

If parahormone is over-produced and hyperparathyroidism results, blood calcium rises and mineral salts are not laid down in the bones, so they become soft, fragile and deformed. The thyroid-parathyroid complex has a resonant interaction with the respiratory and skeletal systems. Through calcium ion modulation the nerves and muscles are made more or less sensitive to stimuli.

Psychologically our conceptual mind provides a framework and organizes the processing of the images which guide our life and enables us to manifest as a social being. When mental arousal is low we do not function very well. As arousal increases we reach an optimum range when we are most efficient and feel most comfortable. As we get more aroused we become confused and less efficient. When we are young, simple things occupy our attention. As we learn and grow we integrate our experience and can handle more and more complex tasks. When life gets boring or tedious we need to seek new challenges to arouse our minds optimally. If we do not, we end up like a zombie. If the challenges are too great and we cannot handle them we may opt for a nervous breakdown. The normal development process moves through periods of assimilating new experiences into established frameworks followed by times of apparent chaos as our minds are reorganized to accomodate a new mental framework. It is important to appreciate the special times when you think 'I don't know anything anymore'. Live with it and love yourself. The confusion will pass in a while. Resorting to the 'uppers' and 'downers' of psychoactive drugs is not an optimal solution. Your mind will sort itself out and regular yoga practice will help you through.

The thymus

The chemical equivalent of the Anahata Chakra, the thymus is an irregularly shaped organ, located just behind the breast bone. Fairly large at birth, it continues to grow until puberty, by which time it normally weighs 30-40g. In early life it is pinkish-grey in colour but later becomes yellowish through replacement by fat.

The thymus is the master gland of the immune system. It is the 'ego' of our body, labelling everything in our system 'me' and attacking anything that is labelled 'not me' through the lymphocytes. The thymus secretes a number of polypeptide hormones including thymosin which gives T-lymphocytes the capacity to produce their natural drugs such as interferon that act directly on toxic invaders to protect the body. If the thymus is underactive we are prey to all kinds of body invaders. If we do not possess sufficient ego strength we tend to over-react to psycho-social pressures. This results in very high secretion of corticosteroids. High concentrations of corticosterone damages thymic tissue and lymphocytes.

Over activity of the thymus results in our immune system attacking its own body just as some people do violence to themselves when their aggression turns back on them. Our own self-preservation system works against us to produce autoimmune diseases such as rheumatoid arthritis, multiple sclerosis or cancer. Many of the symptoms associated with virus infection are not due to the presence of the virus but to the immune response. Allergies are due in part to an exaggerated immune response.

It is not the environmental situation as such that causes stress, it is our reaction to it. Whilst the thymus remains healthy we remain young, but the thymus is one of the first body tissues to break down in senile decay, and when it does so the rest of the body soon follows. Yogis remain youthful.

In yoga practice we expand our self image (pranayama) to include others. Whatever we accept as 'self' is preserved. Whatever is rejected as 'alien' is attacked and destroyed or banished from our territory. Cardiovascular function is in resonance with this system and it is not without good psychosomatic foundation that we need to open our hearts to others.

The pancreas

The pancreas (nabhi) is the endocrine equivalent of the Manipura Chakra. It is a large organ about 5-5½ in. in length and shaped rather like a Conference pear. The pancreas produces chemicals which influence the stomach and the liver, although only 1 or 2 per cent of the pancreas acts as an endocrine organ. The Islets of Langerhans, which are scattered throughout the entire pancreas, produce glucagon and insulin. Glucagon promotes the breakdown

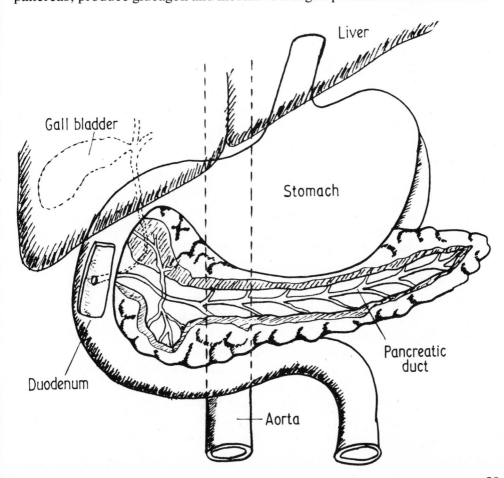

of glycogen in glucose—simple sugars which are used by the body tissues. The body normally stores glucose in great chains as glycogen. It reduces glycogen breakdown to glucose in the liver and increases glycogen formation from glucose particularly in the muscles, thus lowering the blood sugar level. Reduced insulin formation may result in diabetes melitis, which produces progressive drowsiness leading to coma and finally death as a result of the muscles being unable to use glucose efficiently. Excessive secretion of insulin results in hyperinsulinism, a low blood-sugar condition in which the metabolism of the nervous tissue is impaired and giddiness and convulsions may result.

Metabolism means 'change' and pancreas malfunction indicates an inability to handle change in life. It can be your failure to create change which disturbs you, or conversely it can be your inability to cope with the changes going on around you. Yogis tend to be able to handle change both within and around themselves.

The major role of insulin is in differentiating cells. Insulin exerts an important influence on the way cells grow and take on special functions.

The adrenals

Representing the Svasdithana Chakra, there are two adrenal glands in the body, one just above and slightly in front of each kidney (vrikkau), (hence the name adrenals, which means near or next to the kidney). They look rather yellow in colour and usually weigh 3-5g. The outer surface of the gland is called the cortex, which means 'rind' and the inner part is called the medulla, which means 'marrow'. The medulla is essentially an extension of the sympathetic nervous system. It produces adrenalin which is associated with the psychological experience of fear, and noradrenalin, which is associated with anger. These hormones appear to help the organism cope with short-term crises. Through their effect on the sympathetic nervous system the heart rate is increased, the blood pressure rises and blood is diverted from the visceral organs to the muscles and the brain. Glycogen stores in the liver are released to provide glucose as fuel for the body.

The cortex contains three different groups of cells arranged in layers, and these probably produce three different hormones. The first is called aldostrone which has a salt-retaining action. The second—hydrocortisone—has a sugar-producing action. It causes the body to start breaking down its own protein to produce glucose, this being one of the effects of fasting on the body. Androgen, the third hormone means 'male-producer', and it is responsible for the growth of hair on the limbs, chest, lower abdominal wall, armpits and the face. It also causes recession of the hair at the temples and through producing changes in the larynx, causes the voice to deepen. Androgen also produces acne and emotionally it induces a tendency to become more aggressive.

60

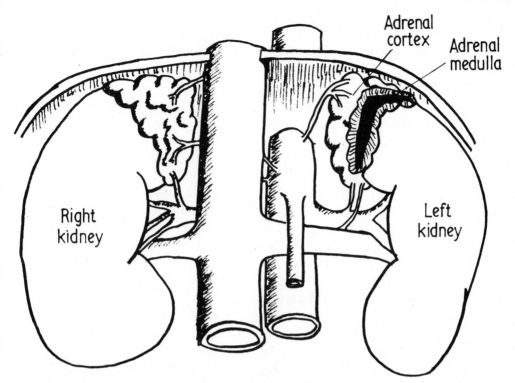

Right kidney

Left kidney

Adrenal cortex

Adrenal medulla

Hormone secretion in the adrenal glands follows a twenty-four hour rhythm, as do most processes in the body. The adrenal glands are associated with the social response and with the following functions:

1   Control of oxidation of all body cells, regulating

    a nerve energy (oxidation of phosphorus in the brain and nerve tissue)

    b physical energy and heat (oxidation of carbon in the muscles)

    c special organ function (oxidation in liver & kidneys)

    d life of every body cell (impossible without oxidation)

2   Control tone of

    a voluntary muscles (bodily strength)

    b heart muscles (circulation, blood pressure)

    c involuntary muscles (peristalsis, uterine tone)

3   Control of number of circulating blood cells, red and white

4   Control of blood clotting (probably also assisted by parathyroids)

5   Control of degree of body immunity

6   Control of the rate of red cell sedimentation

The gonads

The gonads are associated with the Muladhara Chakra. From the moment of conception the human body is continuously developing and sexual differentiation slowly takes place during this process. Hormones determine whether you are developed as a biological male, a biological female, or as sometimes happens, with aspects of both sexes. Oestrogenic hormones stimulate the development and maintenance of female sex characteristics and inhibit the development of male characteristics. Androgenic hormones stimulate the reverse process. Hormones do not create organs, they simply modify pre-existing characteristics. In order to have a powerful effect, hormones must be present in a certain concentration. Both oestrogen and androgen are present in both sexes and the degree of maleness and femaleness is dependent upon the relative amounts of each.

The sex glands have two functions; they produce and release gametes and also secrete hormones. Male glands—called testes—are composed of semineferous tubles which are concerned with the creation of sperm cells and the interstitial cells which develop hormones. Spermatozoa are formed continuously in very large numbers from puberty right into old age. In an early stage of fetal development the testes are located in the abdominal cavity, moving down as development takes place until they finally enter a sac called the scrotum just before birth. Sometimes this descent does not take place, resulting in infertility as sperm cells cannot be produced in the high temperature of the body but require the slightly lower temperature outside the main body.

The hormones of the testes are associated with physical aggression, and this knowledge has been used effectively for thousands of years to tame both animals and men by castration. Imbalanced hormone production results in male baldness and it is significant that most yogis maintain a full head of hair all their life.

The female ovaries are greyish-pink in colour and each weighs 5-7g. They have an inner surface which forms the germinal layer and an outer zone where the follicles contain the ova. The primary follicles change into growing follicles which develop into mature follicles. The mature follicle then ruptures, liberating the ovum which passes with follicular fluid into the abdominal cavity. This process is called ovulation and it occurs in a biocycle of about twenty-eight days, commencing at puberty and continuing until menopause.

At the time of conception approximately 200 million sperm cells rush towards the one ovum, but only one sperm cell actually unites with the ovum to fertilize it. The rest disintegrate. During pregnancy, a number of

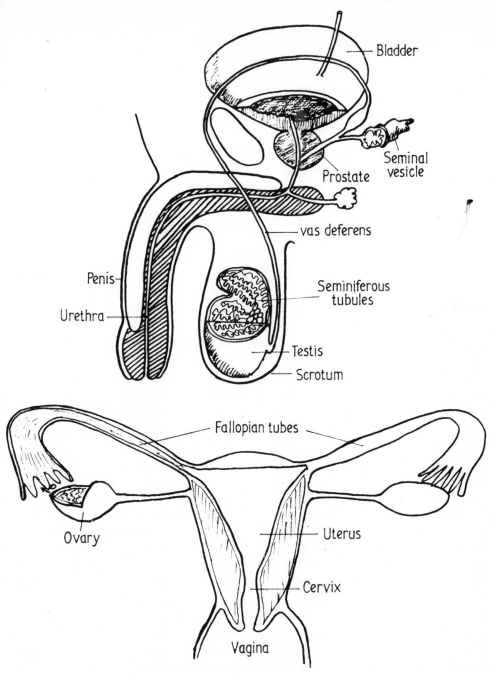

important changes take place in the female. The growing placenta acts as an additional endocrine organ producing oestrogen and progesterone which, amongst other things, help develop the breasts.

The sex glands may be thought of as playing an important role in species preservation, as opposed to the adrenal glands which are more concerned with personal preservation.

6 Akash and Prana

The chakra system represents the universe of form and matter. Form, matter and energy are interchangeable, being but different states of the same thing. All energy is known as Prana in yoga, and all form is known as Akash, which is manifested through the power of Prana. Akash comes from the word *Kash* meaning 'radiant energy'; Akash is space as the mother of form.

Nuclear force, electromagnetic force, weak interaction force, gravity, bio-energy, and psychic-energy are all forms of Prana. Particles, atoms, molecules, cells, animals, men, planets and suns are all forms of Akash. Just as nuclear force is obtained through splitting of the nucleus of an atom, so Prana is obtained through the splitting of Akash; and just as the energy of an atomic nucleus and the nucleus itself are inseparable, so Prana and Akash are inseparable. All matter is created from Akash and we will return to it. The universe is a universe of vibration and cycles. All is composed of limited manifestation and unlimited non-manifestation. Consciousness is unlimited but it can only manifest itself by working through limitation. Consciousness is like a television programme which is present everywhere in the electromagnetic ocean and manifests according to our personal tuning through our body, which acts as a television set.

Kumbhak and Prana

According to yoga, consciousness which manifests through our body, ie through our personality, is like a pot which has both air inside and outside it. The word for pot in Sanskrit is *kumbhak* and Pranayama is sometimes called Kumbhak. In yoga the air inside is called Antar Kumbhak and the air outside Bahya Kumbhak. The change from Antar Kumbhak to Bahya Kumbhak is called Rechakh, while the reverse change from Bahya Kumbhak to Antar Kumbhak is called Purakh. All the rhythmic cycles of the universe are composed of these four stages—Antar Kumbhak, Rechakh, Bahya Kumbhak and Purakh. The most familiar of these cycles is that of our own breathing. Our respiratory cycle has four stages breathing in, Purakh; holding breath in, Antar Kumbhak, breathing air out, Rechakh; holding breath out, Bahya Kumbhak. As long as this cycle is repeated we live in the body, when the cycle is finished we are pronounced dead. Thus control of this cycle is mastery of life.

By expanding our personal energy and control we may grow. Everything in the universe is either growing or dying. The process of death is called entropy in physics and is seen as the dissolution of form. The diametrically opposed process is called negative entropy. It is the life process, the manifestation of form, which is known about and maintained by communication. The process of communication starts from Self, enters into vibration and matter, and finishes represented to Self. I am the beginning and the end is a cosmic statement which describes communication. Perfect communication is called health, wholeness and yoga, whereas breakdown of communication is called disease. For perfect health, physical and biological, psychological and spiritual, you should practise Pranayama, through which you will be able to control your energy ups and downs, and make energy available for use when you need it. Through Pranayama personal energy is transformed into cosmic energy, enabling you to transform your personal identity with the limited ego into cosmic identity.

The life force—Prana—is manifested as motion and sensation. All sensation and perception is represented at the biological level by the nervous system, while the source of all motion in the body is the heart, and communication of energy is maintained by the circulatory system assisted by the respiratory system.

Prana has five divisions in the body:

Prana   The main function of prana is to produce motion in the heart and lungs. Its major residence is in the heart and its field of action is the entire body.

Apana   The force by which waste products are removed from the body, as in micturition.

Udana   The force by which we talk, laugh and cry. Its main centre is in the speech areas.

Samana   The force responsible for all metabolic processes. It is centred on the area of the navel.

Vyana   The force by which the cardiovascular system expands and contracts. It prevades the whole body.

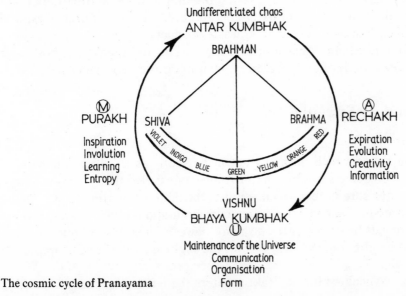

The cosmic cycle of Pranayama

65

The relation of Prana to the body. As well as the five main pranas, five minor pranas govern the following processes: Naga—belching; Kurma—hiccupping; Kukara—yawning; Devadatta—hunger; Dhanayiya—dropping eyelids

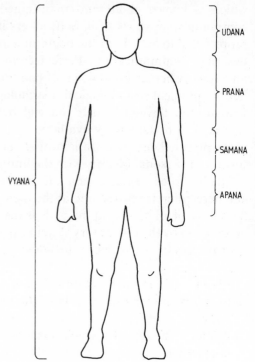

UDANA

PRANA

SAMANA

VYANA

APANA

All life is maintained by the joint action of the external and internal breathing processes. External breathing consists of : ventilation, which includes air both coming in and going out through the respiratory tract; gaseous exchange, which takes place in the lungs; pumping of the heart, which sends the oxygenated blood to every part of the body for internal breathing. Internal breathing takes place in the cells and consists of oxidation and other metabolic processes, and production of carbon dioxide and other waste products.

In order to understand Pranayama and the working of Prana in our bodies we must first make a study of the circulatory, lymphatic and respiratory systems.

The Circulatory System

The heart (Hridaya)

We have two hearts which normally act in harmony as a 170cc, two-cylinder muscular pump. These serve two major routes; one called the systematic circulation, a high pressure system which supplies the main body with blood, and the other a low pressure system - the pulmonary circulation - which passes through the lungs. The left heart is larger and more powerful as it does about six times the work of the right, and this exaggerates the slight skew of the heart to the left side of the body.

Bright red, oxygenated blood (Rakta) enters the left side of the heart and is

66

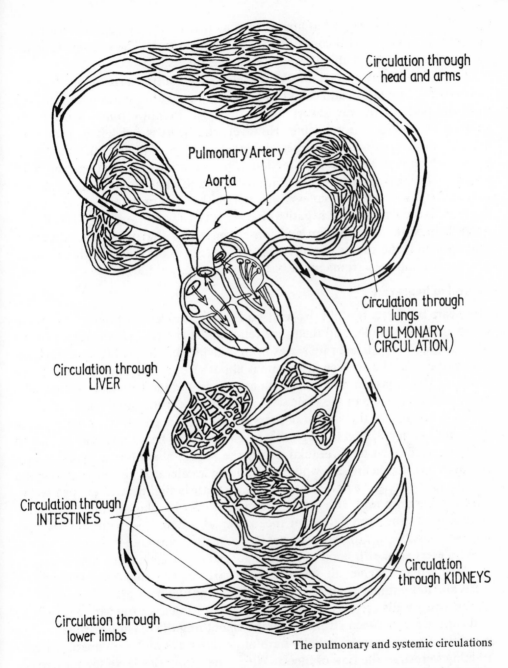

Circulation through
head and arms

Pulmonary Artery

Aorta

Circulation through
lungs
(PULMONARY
CIRCULATION)

Circulation through
LIVER

Circulation through
INTESTINES

Circulation
through KIDNEYS

Circulation through
lower limbs

The pulmonary and systemic circulations

pumped out through the aorta. The aorta is about 1in across initially but soon divides into smaller and smaller branches called arteries (dhamanis) and arterioles and finally into capillaries (srotamsi). As the blood gives up its oxygen to the cells (dhatus) of the body it gradually turns dark red. The blood is recollected through venules which join to form the veins (siras) which return the blood through the right side of the heart to the pulmonary (lung) circulation, where it regains its bright red appearance as it takes up oxygen. Returning to the left side of the heart it continues its ceaseless journey. The shortest time for the blood to circulate is about twenty-seven heartbeats.

The heart is a very special kind of muscle, for it contracts rhythmically without nervous stimulation and can keep on beating even after it has been removed from the body. This was always known in yoga literature but was originally laughed at by Western medicine. However, the heart is not left to beat haphazardly but is conducted by a specially sensitive piece of tissue called the 'pacemaker' which is situated at the junction of the superior vena cava and the right atrium. The heart movement is initiated through changes of potassium and sodium ions. Ions are molecules which have either lost or gained electrons and therefore have a positive or negative charge. It is known in yoga that it is Prana which brings about ionisation and ion changes and that thus it is ultimately Prana which is the source of movement and energy in the body. With each beat the heart radiates electromagnetic pulses to every part of the body.

Control of heart rate

The heart beat is a twofold process; both the ventricles contract in the phase which is called systole, and then they relax whilst the two atria contract in the diastole phase. The heart rate varies from individual to individual and throughout the day, but the average heart rate is about seventy beats per minute. There is a general decrease in rate from birth to old age and the female heart normally beats a little faster than the male. Adjacent to the carotid sinus, just below the ear on either side of the neck, is a pressure-sensitive nerve. It is a branch of the ninth cranial nerve, and through this mechanism the heart rate may be slowed or accelerated. The tenth cranial nerve, the vagus, also plays a major role in slowing down the heart rate while sympathetic accelerator nerves tend to speed it up by influencing the pacemaker. The heart rate is slightly affected by psychological experience and with a little practice it may be placed under deliberate control. It may be slowed down or speeded up at will and, with greater practice, it is even possible to stop the heart beat for extended periods.[1]

With every stroke 70-80ml of blood is pushed out of each side of the heart. By the time a man reaches his seventies his heart has beaten some 3,000 million times and has pumped over 420,000 metric tons of blood.

The artery walls are elastic, enabling them to stretch a little with each stroke and contract in between strokes, thereby smoothing the diastolic pressure. The arterioles (small arteries) usually have muscular walls and are capable of contracting to restrict the flow of blood. Where the capillaries leave them there is a ring of muscle called a sphincter which acts rather like a tap. There are about 68,000sq ft of blood capillaries in the adult body and it is across this surface that the exchange of materials between the blood and the tissues takes place. The total cross-section of the capillaries is some nine hundred times that of the aorta, and without these little taps to control the blood flow standing upright would be most hazardous as blood would quickly drain from our heads and we

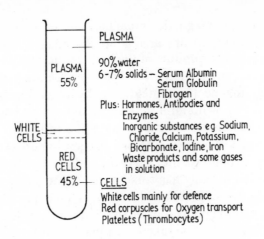

PLASMA

90% water
6-7% solids — Serum Albumin
                Serum Globulin
                Fibrogen
Plus: Hormones, Antibodies and
      Enzymes
      Inorganic substances eg Sodium,
        Chloride, Calcium, Potassium,
        Bicarbonate, Iodine, Iron
      Waste products and some gases
        in solution

CELLS
White cells mainly for defence
Red corpuscles for Oxygen transport
Platelets (Thrombocytes)

The composition of the blood

might well bulge at the ankles. Capillary circulation directed by vyana may be controlled precisely with a little training, although it is only recently that western medicine has realised this.

Blood

An average sized man contains about 5 l of blood. At the biological level the blood has three major functions: firstly, it conveys water, food, oxygen, and all forms of Prana to the entire body; secondly, it removes waste products and all forms of apana through the kidneys, liver and lungs; thirdly, it distributes heat and agents to combat disease and injury, and provides a communication network for hormonal control of the body processes.

Blood is about 55 per cent plasma—a straw-coloured liquid—and 45 per cent cells. 90 per cent of the plasma is water, about 7 per cent is composed of various proteins and the rest is made up of salts. It contains hormones and traces of many other substances, eg waste products.

Blood cells (Rakta) can be divided into two groups: red and white. The so-called red blood cells, which carry haemoglobin, are not true cells as they have lost their nucleus, although they do begin their life complete when they are produced in the bone marrow (majja). In yoga one of haemoglobin's most important properties is the magnetic change which it undergoes when it takes up oxygen. If a tube of venous blood is suspended vertically between the poles of an electromagnet it appears to get heavier when the field is switched on, but after the blood has taken up oxygen it gets lighter instead. As there is a greater amount of oxygenated blood on the left side of the body, owing to the action of the left heart in receiving and pumping bright red blood, and a greater amount of deoxygenated blood on the right side, the magnetic field of the body is asym-

69

metrical. This left/right magnetic imbalance is made use of in many yogic practices, eg pranayama, janusirasana, gomukhasana.

The most significant end-product of the bodily processes and the end-product of food in the body is hydrogen ions. The hydrogen ion is a hydrogen atom which has lost its surrounding electronic field. The hydrogen ion is simply a proton. The proton is the basis of life and may be thought of as positive electricity or 'proticity'. Hydrogen ions in the blood lower the affinity of haemoglobin for oxygen. This promotes the release of any oxygen bound to haemoglobin and aids the uptake of carbon dioxide. Oxygen tends to be taken up by a haemoglobin molecule which already has some oxygen, and prefers the haemoglobin with more oxygen to haemoglobin with less. It is a good example of the biblical parable of the rich and the poor. 'For he that hath, to him shall be given, and he that hath not, from him shall be taken even that which he hath.' Through these means oxygen is taken to the body tissues and carbon dioxide is removed.

The white blood cells (leucocytes) are less numerous and there is normally about one white cell for every 600 red cells. Of these about two thirds are granular leucocytes and the remaining third are agranular. The majority of the granular leucocytes are called neutrophils. They do not swim in the blood but crawl, rather like an amoeba, and so they need surfaces to move along. In the blood vessels they hug the walls whilst the red cells continuously rotating remain in the centre of the stream. They are the 'commandos' of the body and their life expectancy is short. When a foreigner such as a bacterium invades they are the first to go into action. A neutrophil may 'eat' as many as fifty bacteria before being killed itself, depending on the nature of the bacteria. At the site of a major battle millions of dead leucocytes collect as pus.

Most of the agranular leucocytes are called lymphocytes and are formed in the lymphatic system which is examined below in more detail. The number of white cells in the blood of healthy persons varies with the number of sunspots. There is an exact monthly correlation of the leucocyte content in the blood and the sun's rotational activity.

A third element in the blood is known as a platelet. These are formed in the bone marrow and are smaller and even less of a true cell than the red erithrocytes. They are more numerous than white but less numerous than red corpuscles and are called thrombocytes because they play an important role in blood clotting.

The Lymphatic and the Immune System

The water in the body is distributed between three compartments separated by membranes which regulate fluid transport in both directions across their surfaces. The first compartment is the tubular system of the blood stream, where the water first accumulates from food and drink which has been taken. The water, with a small percentage of proteins, salts and lymphocytes, diffuses across the blood vessel membrane into the second compartment. This interstitial fluid is called lymph (rasa) and surrounds each cell as a go-between between the

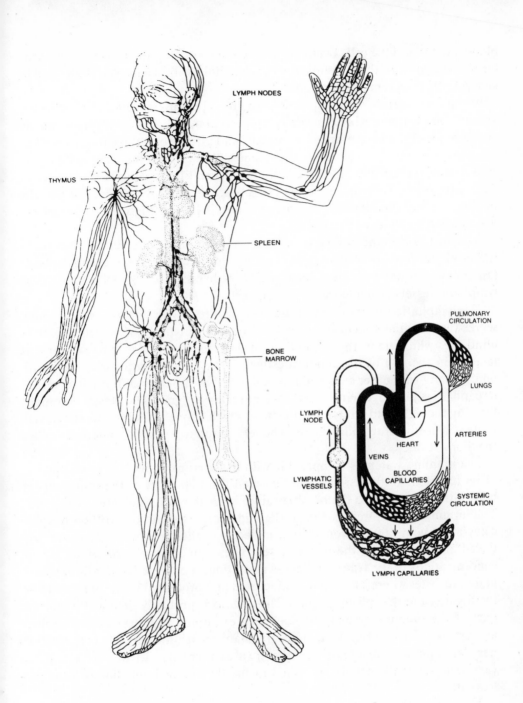

LYMPH NODES

THYMUS

SPLEEN

BONE
MARROW

PULMONARY
CIRCULATION

LUNGS

LYMPH
NODE

ARTERIES

HEART

VEINS

LYMPHATIC
VESSELS

BLOOD
CAPILLARIES

SYSTEMIC
CIRCULATION

LYMPH CAPILLARIES

The lymphatic system

blood stream and the cell. Lymph is assisted in its circulation by general muscular movement. The third compartment is the fluid within each cell itself, and in general this fluid remains constant.

Initial dehydration shows up first in the blood compartment and later in the second compartment which normally contains about 81. When this happens the capacitance of the membrane is increased, and after two or three days of continued abstinence from water the body becomes so dry that it builds up a high surface charge of electricity. In this condition you can lift up paper through electrostatic attraction. Dehydration often takes place during yoga practice, especially in Yoga Nidra (Chapter 14), and the skin obtains a very high electrical charge, owing to the build up of Prana.

It is most important to keep up a good water intake during Hatha Yoga practice or kidney and other damage may result. Prana requires water, and the body (annamaya kosha) may be thought of as rather like a wet-cell battery. The lymphatic vessels are called srotas in Sanskrit.

The lymphatic system is a vascular system fitted with one-way valves which serves the immune system in our body. The tree of lymphatic vessels begins as blind sacs which lie in the tissue fluid of deep tissues, organs and skin and as lacteals in the villi of the small intestine. These collect lymphocytes and antibodies along with other cells and molecules and the interstitial fluid. The vessels or capillaries join together to form larger and larger lymphatic vessels eventually forming the right and left lymphatic ducts which empty back into the subclavian veins just behind the collar bone. The left lymphatic duct is sometimes called the thoracic duct.

The immune system is comparable with the nervous system in the complexity of its function. Both systems are dispersed through most of the tissues of the body although owing to the blood/brain barrier they seem to avoid each other. The immune system weighs nearly 1kg and contains about one trillion lymphocytes and about 100 million trillion molecules called antibodies that are produced and secreted by the lymphocytes. These lymphocytes are found in high concentrations in the lymph nodes—way-stations along the lymphatic vessels—and at the sites where they are manufactured and processed in the bone marrow, the thymus and the spleen (plijha). The thymus is probably the most important part of the immune system and has been examined in more detail elsewhere as part of the endocrine system. More than ten trillion (10,000,000,000,000) new lymphocytes are created in the thymus every day of our lives and the vast majority of these cells are killed in the thymus or immediately after they leave it.

There are large numbers of lymph nodes which serve to remove foreign matter, such as bacteria and dead red corpuscles, from the lymph and thus prevent it entering the blood. These lymph nodes are found in high concentration in certain areas of the body such as the neck, the groin and the tonsils. It is useful to note that the lymph carries fats, obtained mainly from the small intestines, that would be harmful to the red corpuscles in the blood.

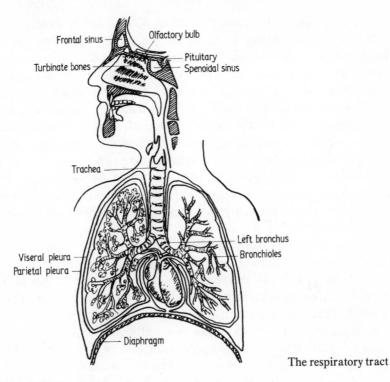

The frontal sinus, Olfactory bulb, Turbinate bones, Pituitary, Spenoidal sinus, Trachea, Left bronchus, Bronchioles, Viseral pleura, Parietal pleura, Diaphragm

The respiratory tract

The Respiratory System

If we breathe in through the mouth (mukha) we lose a great deal of valuable effects and gain a number of unwanted problems. Normally, air enters the respiratory tract through the nostrils and all coarse particles are strained out of the air by the hairs around the entrance. Inside the nose (nasa) the direction of air flow changes to the horizontal and air has to pass along curving channels. Small particles that may have eluded the hairy traps do not change direction easily and are caught on one or another of the many projections. Four pairs of hollows called sinuses lead off from the nasal passages. These are located in the frontal, ethmoid, sphenoid and maxillary bones and are of major importance in yoga.

The sinuses and the entire respiratory tract are lined with ciliated epithilial cells (kala). This lining is kept moist by the mucus (kapha) which is secreted from goblet cells. All the cilia beat in rhythm towards the exits to remove irritating particles and mucus. This epithilial lining is studded with nerve endings which lead back to the brain and particularly to the hypothalamus.

Air passing through the nasal passages is thus cleaned, warmed and moistened. The air continues back and down the windpipe which branches into two tubes called bronchi, each leading to a separate lung (phuphusa). The bronchi subdivide into smaller bronchioles and each tiny bronchioli ends in a number of little air sacs called alveoli. There are about 600 million alveoli and their total surface area is twenty-five times that of the whole body. The lungs are covered

73

with an airtight membrane called the pleura which secretes a serous fluid to lubricate the breathing movements. Through expanding the rib cage and a lowering of the diaphragm (peshimukhadwayi) the pressure in the lungs is reduced and air is drawn in. This is inspiration, which also assists the return of venous blood to the heart. A little extra air may be drawn into the lungs by raising the shoulder up and back but this is a most uneconomical action. Breathing out, or expiration, is principally accomplished by muscular relaxation although forced expiration can be produced by muscle contraction if necessary. Coughing, sneezing, laughing, crying, sighing and yawning are all modified respiratory movements and are considered to be controlled by particular pranas in yoga.

Every inspiration is accompanied by a marked change in the electrical potential of the skin which can be an increase of a decrease in the order of 10 millivolts DC.

The total lung capacity has been estimated to be about 5.51. Tidal air is the amount of air breathed in and out of the lungs during normal respiration and is usually about 0.51. With forced inspiration another 21 can be breathed in and with a little effort something like 1.51 can be breathed out. The residual air, ie what is left in the lungs even after maximum expiration, amounts to about 1.51. The biggest breath you can take is usually called your vital capacity and averages 3.5-4.01 although individuals differ quite a lot in their capacity.

Your breathing rate varies considerably according to what you are doing physically and psychically. At rest, the rate is usually about fifteen breaths per minute. The rate and depth of breathing is controlled by respiratory centres in the central nervous system which integrate information from mechanical and chemical receptors. Essential control of the respiratory centre may be exercised deliberately but is biologically determined by hydrogen ions—proticity—in the cerebro-spinal fluid. Increased carbon dioxide in the arterial blood reduces the arterial proticity; this changes the cerebro-spinal fluid proticity which in turn influences the respiratory centres in the medulla oblongata.

Generally, we do not breathe evenly through both nostrils. On average we tend to breathe for an hour predominantly through the left nostril then, after breathing through both during a short change-over period, we breathe through the right for about an hour. This changing of nostril dominance follows a pattern which varies with the time of day and with the time of the month. In yoga variations from the ideal pattern of nostril breathing can be used for accurate diagnosis and prognosis. It is even claimed that the day and time of one's death can be predicted.[2] Breathing through the left nostril has a relaxing, cholinergic effect on the body. It has been shown that ESP capability increases significantly when breathing through the left nostril as compared with the right nostril or the mouth. Breathing through the right nostril produces an adrenergic effect.

The air we breathe contains ions which have a very remarkable effect on plants, animals and men. The concentrations of ions and the ratio of positive to negative may change considerably. In modern city life man usually encounters very low concentration of ions and a preponderance of positive over negative

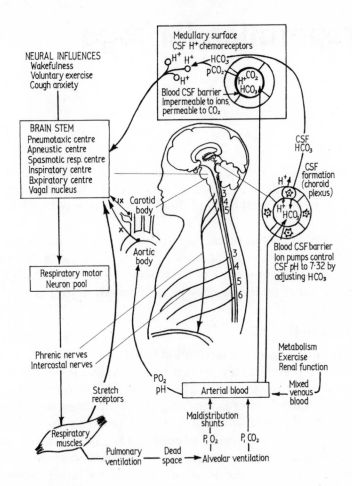

Nervous centres of breathing

small air ions. Higher concentrations of ions are found in unpolluted country spaces, while the proportion of negative ions increases, particularly in mountainous areas. Basically, negative ions have a beneficial effect on the body. They tend to slow down respiration, lower blood pressure, increase the action of cilia in the respiratory passages and bring a feeling of mental alertness and general well-being. On the other hand positive ions slow down the ciliary beat and produce contracture of the smooth muscle of the air passages. In general, ion depletion leads to discomfort, inertia, and lassitude, and loss of mental and physical efficiency, while an increase of ions relieves the pain of burns and promotes body growth and restoration. Negative ions significantly help learning and reduce anxiety whereas we tend to become aggressive in positive ions conditions.

Oxygen ions are negative, carbon dioxide ions are positive and water ions may be either positive or negative. Relatively, the air breathed out is positively charged and the air breathed in negatively charged. Considerable use is made of these factors in yoga breathing techniques and in other practices.

7 Preparation for Yoga

At the beginning of this book it was pointed out that yoga practice can be seen as the positive half of life. Thus yoga is not a Friday night or Sunday morning practice, it is an entire way of life and should occupy twenty-four hours of every day.

There are many factors to be carefully considered if the maximum benefit is to be gained from the deliberate practice of Hatha Yoga. At the base of all yoga practice is the constant observance of the yamas and niyamas which were examined earlier. Nevertheless, the psychological approach to yoga is also supremely important.

Preparing your mind

The dominating psychological contribution to life is expectancy. For example, it has been shown that even highly trained scientists tend to get the results from their experiment that they expect and because of this the results of different researchers can be quite contradictory. Again, it has been demonstrated that whilst 70 per cent of people find that morphine relieves pain symtoms, half of this effect is very probably the result of expectancy, and sugar pills might prove an equally effective substitute as long as the patient is unaware of the deception.

Our experience of life and the results of our work are largely governed by our expectancy. Our very sensations are directed by our expectations; for example, many people have drunk a cup of coffee believing it to be tea! Even our intelligence appears to be affected by expectation, and it appears that children will grow brighter and become more creative simply because they are expected to do so. Certainly our progress in yoga is very much determined by our own expectancy.

Expectancy is not simply wishful thinking but a deep suggestion to our imagination that a certain result will occur. The degree of fulfilment which we get in life will vary according to the strength of our expectations. Ordinary thinking is a low-level process and is basically the regurgitation and manipulation of our memory traces. Yogis do very little of this kind of thinking. Their minds are engaged at the deeper level of the imagination, for they know that it is our imagination which makes us what we are and thus the master of the imagination is a master of life.

The imagination is like a garden. Any seed which is planted in it and nourished will grow, while ideas and images which are not required have to be weeded out or deprived of nutrition so that they die away. Weeds can easily overgrow the garden and choke the useful plants if they are left unchecked. The aim of the yamas is to attack these weeds while the niyamas nourish the useful plants so that they may later bear fruit.

Therefore the first preparation for yoga and for life is to imagine clearly the results that you wish to obtain. Secondly you must realise that you will undoubtedly attain these goals. The universe is waiting to give you everything you need; it exists only to serve the Self. It is natural to doubt this but if you do not accept it you will slow up your progress considerably. Life is not a hard fight for survival nor is progress in yoga something which must be strived for. Expect success in your yoga practice, but do not be disturbed and disappointed by any apparent lack of progress. You are very near to yourself and will not be able to see the fundamental changes taking place in your life. Perhaps others around you will notice the difference before you do. Your teacher will observe your progress knowingly, having been through the same experience himself. You may at first believe that it is the people around you who are changing, like sitting on a train and suddenly noticing that the station is moving, but soon you realise that it is you who are making the real progress. As you make progress your smaller problems disappear and bigger ones present themselves. The bigger your problems are the more progress the universe expects you to make, and thus you will never get a problem that you cannot handle.

When you discover that you are making real progress you must then realise that countless others have done the same and so do not allow yourself to become self-opinionated or arrogant. Any feelings of superiority simply indicate that you have not yet learned the first basic lesson of yoga practice—that all is Self. Looking at your own progress and feeling pleased about it is a waste of time and a side-tracking temptation. Let others assess your progress if they wish, but do not boast of your achievements or acclaim your experiences yourself as you will find that this removes the likelihood of further progress.

There is no greater rule in life than to do your absolute best and always do what you believe to be right at the time. If your behaviour proves to be wrong later, learn from it but do not dwell on it. You should always be totally concerned with manifesting what is good and right, but at the same time you must not be tempted to fight evil and unrighteousness. It is better to fight the 'good' fight and assert the positive than to occupy yourself with the negative and fail to supply the positive.

Make it a way of life to observe yourself, for by being aware of your behaviour you will be your own guru and will learn things from yourself that you did not know you knew. By being fully aware of other people everybody will be your guru and by being completely aware of your environment the entire universe will be your teacher. By attending fully to everything you do, you will not only be far more successful in the world but you will find even the most boring jobs enjoyable. Through concentration on your life you will achieve fulfilment and your ego will disappear taking with it all your desires. As your desires disappear, the pleasures and pains, the ups and downs, the opposites of life, will fade away and the true happiness of fulfilment will pervade your being. The eternal truth that all is Self will shine through you to light the way for others to follow.

Environmental considerations

Everything around you presents suggestions to your imagination. As you affect your environment, so your environment, particularly your own room, is a description of your own mind. The political and social processes of today are an accurate description of the mind of man at the present stage. Mankind has not even the ability to govern himself peacefully, and wars, conflicts and tensions are the content of our news programmes. The 4,000 million people alive today are blaming others for the state of the world.

Look at your friends and associates carefully. As a group they are probably a fairly good description of yourself, for socially, birds of a feather do flock together. It is easy to be attracted to places and activities which will dissipate your energies and distract you from your personal intention to discover the real nature of yourself and to manifest it. Observe moths and flies attracted to a flame at night. They fly straight into the flame and perish. There are genuine people who search for Self through drugs, but we have never met anybody who, having had more than the slightest contact with drugs, has fully attained the goal of self-discovery. Many famous writers on the subject of self-discovery are themselves psychologically confused although they are taken as positive examples by their readers who do not know them personally. Do not fool yourself and follow the worst examples but associate yourself with the best exponents of what you are aiming for. If you read books on personal growth and yoga, read those which are written by people who actually practise what they preach. Nobody can be an authority on a subject if he is not himself an example of what he advocates.

It is a great advantage to select a sympathetic environment in which to live. You have the power to change your environment, so exercise it. If you are doing a job which makes it very difficult to practise yoga, then you can choose between the job and personal fulfillment. It is possible to do a job or plan a career which is absolutely consonant with yoga principles if you really want to. You may wish to deny this, but it will only be a psychological defence which will come between you and your real Self.

Look at your room. Is it tidy and clean? Is it colourful or dull, harmonious or ugly? Remember, it is a self-description, if it is the room in which you are going to practise yoga exercises, make it suitable. If you have a spare room to devote totally to yoga practice so much the better, but if not, optimise your surroundings anyway.

At first, it is better to have as few distractions around as possible, or your mind will wander and you will lose your concentration. Without proper concentration your work will be near useless, at best a waste of time, and possibly even damaging.

Colour affects us a great deal, so choose the colour of the room carefully.

Make sure you have room to work in and that the room is clean and dust-free. The floor should be even or some asanas will be very difficult to perform. It is not good to practise yoga in direct sunlight, even though it seems a very healthy thing to do. Ensure that the temperature is maintained at a reasonable level (somewhere between 70 and 80°F). If it is too cool your body will lose a lot of its suppleness and you are highly likely to cause yourself some physical damage. It is good to practise asanas and Pranayama in very light clothing or even in the nude if suitable. Heavy clothing will get in the way.

It is a good idea to keep a special mat for practice of asanas and other practical techniques. As you will probably place your face flat on your mat quite frequently it is essential to keep it clean. Certain exercises will be difficult and dangerous if your mat is not large enough and does not have a non-slip backing. A mat just a little longer than your own height is best and it should be about 30in wide. Again, choose a mat with harmonious colours. If you only practise yoga on that mat it will soon build up an association in your mind which will help put you in a yogic frame of mind every time you sit on it. Traditionally, yogis have mats made of doe or tiger skin.

Timing

Timing of a practical session is very important. It is most unadvisable to attempt any practical work on a stomach that is not fairly empty. At least two hours should have elapsed after a light snack before practice and much longer if the meal was at all heavy. Although you will probably feel hungry anyway, it is advisable to coat the stomach with food after a session as it is likely that plenty of digestive juices will have been manufactured during Hatha Yoga practice.

The best times of day for practising yoga are first thing in the morning or the middle of the evening, although mid-morning and mid-afternoon are also possible times. In the morning you will be stiffer and evening practice has the advantage of a supple body, but in the morning your mind will probably be fresher and you will get more out of your session. It is better to keep the same time aside every day for your yoga practice as this will allow your body's circadian rhythm to adjust satisfactorily.

Women should not practise asanas which place pressure on the abdomen during the first three days of their periods and women who become pregnant should stop practice of asanas and consult their teachers immediately. Proper yoga practice can assist childbirth and give the baby an excellent start in life.

Preparing the body inside and out

Make sure your bowels and bladder are emptied. Students sometimes complain of abdominal pains in the early stages of practice and it is usually because they have not prepared themselves in this way.

You are going to stimulate your bodily organs and pour chemicals into your bloodstream to rebuild and revivify your body, therefore it is important to ensure that your body is clean inside and out. Later when you learn kriyas (special cleansing actions) from your teacher, you may periodically wish to clean your body out very thoroughly. Specialist diet and fasting can also be useful, but in general a thorough bath or shower before yoga practice will be perfectly adequate.

Sankalpa

Before starting any practical session it is useful to get things into perspective. Often in life we become embroiled in the minute and thus do not understand the greater significance of the present. Sankalpa is the technique of reminding yourself about who you are, where you are, the time you are in and the reasons for doing what you are doing.

Composure

To achieve composure sit in a firm, comfortable posture such as the Sukhasana or Padmasana (Chapter 10). Check that your spine is upright and that you are balanced. Now close your eyes and relax from the top of your head downwards: first the face and neck, then the shoulders and arms, finally the chest, abdomen and legs. Check your body for any remaining tensions and relax them. Concentrate on the centre just above and between your eyebrows and let all your thoughts go. Do not try and force them away or they will only come back more insistently; simply let your thoughts go by not attending to them. Concentrate completely on the centre of your forehead. Know that you are about to carry out a programme of work which will be of great benefit to you and that you intend to do it as well as you possibly can. You have the power to change the universe, but you must first change and master yourself.

8 The Surya Namaskar

Generally, the Surya Namaskar may be practised as an independent yoga exercise which removes psychosomatic tensions, improves circulation and stimulates the nervous system through its specific action on the spinal column. It may also be used as a working meditation technique and can help produce great insight into the nature of the universe. Usually the Surya Namaskar is practised before doing asanas as it has a very warming effect on the entire body which is far superior to any athletic limbering up. Practice of the Surya Namaskar will help you achieve in months, results in asanas and other practices which might otherwise take years.

The Surya Namaskar was practised by the ancient rishis on the banks of the sacred river Ganges. *Surya* means 'sun'; *namaskar* is a very beautiful greeting, a recognition of the highest aspect of Self which shines through every being. The Self is the source of the entire universe and the maintainer of every being, as the sun is the source of all life on earth and sustains every creature directly and indirectly. We feed on light and are ultimately made of light. Just as external light on earth is supplied by the sun, so the internal light of consciousness is supplied by the Self. There is no real division between the light which the sun radiates outwards to the ends of the universe and the sun itself, nor is there any real division between the one Self and the consciousness which manifests through all people everywhere.

Traditionally the Surya Namaskar is practised at dawn and is directed towards the sun rising in the east bringing the new day and a fresh opportunity to manifest the good in life.

Method

Position 1   Stand straight with your feet together. Place your palms together touching your chest (1). Concentrate on the sun and imagine its energy pouring into you, filling you with vitality and well-being. Experience the tremendous power of the sun revitalising every cell of your body.

Position 2   Breathe in deeply as you raise your arms and bend backwards from the waist (2).

Position 3   Bend forwards from the hips breathing out slowly. Keeping your legs straight, place your hands flat on the ground by the sides of your feet at shoulder width (3). Place your face on your shins. Keep your hands in the same position during the next few moves.

Position 4   Breathe in and stretch your right leg back so that your foot is at

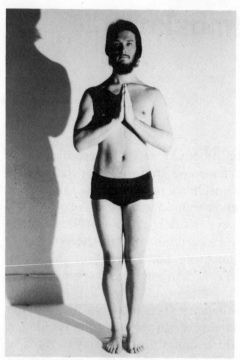

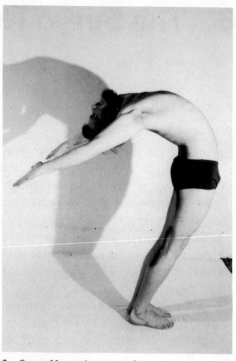

1   Surya Namaskar stage 1

2   Surya Namaskar stage 2

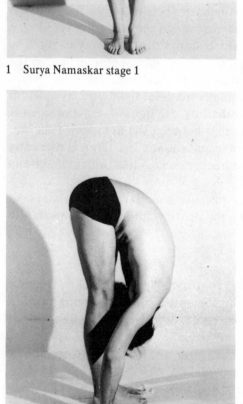

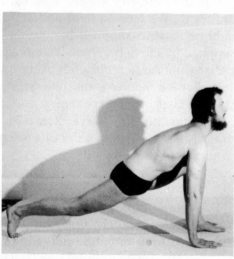

4   Surya Namaskar stage 4

3   Surya Namaskar stage 3

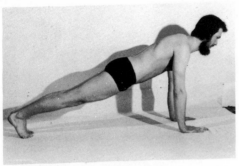

5 Surya Namaskar stage 5

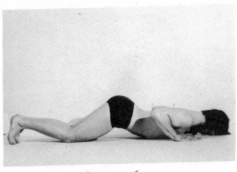

6 Surya Namaskar stage 6

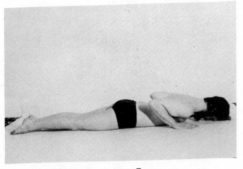

7 Surya Namaskar stage 7

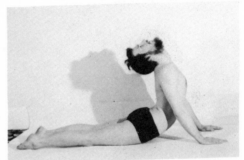

8 Surya Namaskar stage 8

right angles to your leg and resting on its toes. Your left shin should be vertical to the ground and, with your head back, you should be looking towards the horizon (4).

Position 5   Hold your breath as you take your left foot back and place it with the right foot. Maintain your body in a straight line supported only by your toes and hands, which should be in a vertical line. Continue looking at the horizon (5).

Position 6   Still holding your breath, lower your body and rest your toes, knees, chest, palms and forehead on the ground. Your stomach and pelvis should be off the ground and your hands should remain unmoved, but in this position your elbows are bent and your arms should be kept into your sides (6). This position is known as the astanga or eightfold salutation as eight parts of the body are touching the ground.

Position 7   Breathing out, relax flat on the ground (7). Your feet should be resting on the insteps and the hands and arms should remain unmoved from the last position.

Position 8   Breathe in as you raise first your head and then the upper part of your trunk above the navel. Keep your pelvis flat on the ground and relax your bottom and legs. Look back over your body, lightly supporting the top of your body with straightened arms (8).

Position 9   Hold your breath and, bringing your feet flat on to the ground, raise your hips, to form an inverted V shape. Look at your toes (9).

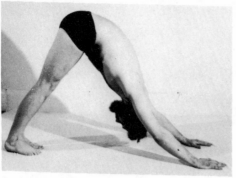

9 Surya Namaskar stage 9

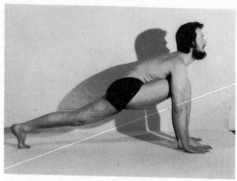

10 Surya Namaskar stage 10

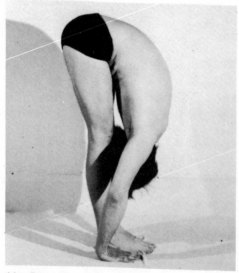

11 Surya Namaskar stage 11

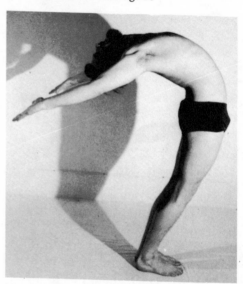

12 Surya Namaskar stage 12

Position 10   Retaining the same breath, bring the right foot forward into the complementary posture to position four (10).

Position 11   Breathe out as you bring the left leg up and place your feet together between your hands. Straighten your legs and place your head on your shins (11).

Position 12   Breathe in as you straighten up from the hips. Bring your arms up, keeping them straight, and stretch them backwards as you bend from the waist. Hold your breath as you look backwards (12).

Position 13   Straighten your body, breathing out as you do so. Bring your arms over your head and, bending your elbows, place your palms together (13). face the horizon ready to breathe in and start a new cycle.

Initially, three repetitions of the cycle is ample. Under normal circumstances you will soon be able to perform the seven or twelve cycles which form an excellent start to a Hatha Yoga programme. Traditionally yogis perform a special number of repetitions, this being 108.

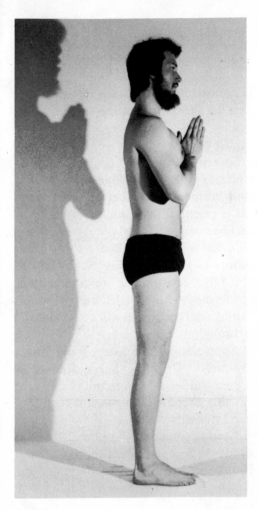

Effects

Position 1   In this position the mind is highly alert and balanced. The bio-energetic currents of the body are able to flow freely with the palms touching and the feet together. Any unevenness of stance, indicating an imbalance of psychosomatic energy, may be consciously corrected.

Position 2   The back is stretched and strengthened, the abdominal muscles stretched and toned up and lung capacity increased.

Position 3   This position is beneficial to the sacral and lower lumbar regions of the spine. It also stretches the hamstrings, lightly massages the abdominal organs and increases the flow of blood to the brain.

Position 4   This tones up the abdomen and pelvis, stretches the thighs and legs, and benefits the base of the spine.

Position 5   The arms, legs and entire trunk are strengthened.

Position 6   This is a unique position in which the natural curvature of the spine is exaggerated thus removing tensions and toning up the entire spine.

Position 7   The entire body is relaxed.

Position 8   The lumbar region of the spine is stretched and toned up and the vagus nerve is stimulated through the slight pressure brought to bear on the carotid sinuses.

Position 9   This position stretches the hamstrings at the back of the knees, strengthens the arms and legs and tones up the sacral area of the spine and the sciatic nerves.

Position 10   The effects are similar to those of position 4.

Position 11   The effects are similar to those of position 3.

Position 12   As with position 2, this produces great abdominal strength.

Position 13   A great many energies and hormones have been released into the body during the previous sequence. It is essential to be highly attentive at this point to balance and control the forces liberated in the body.

As you progress under proper instruction you will discover that as you finish the thirteenth position you will lose all sensory awareness. If there is any lack of concentration at this stage you will probably fall over as though you had fainted, but if your progress has not been hurried, you should have no difficulty in maintaining consciousness and the vertical position. All breathing will cease and the experience of Self—Brahman—will shine through.

When the basic work of Surya Namaskar has been mastered the Surya mantras (sacred thoughts) may be introduced. Thus the Surya Namaskar becomes a multi-levelled exercise of very great value. There are many different mantras which may be incorporated into this exercise and the following are those used by the authors and their advanced students.

The Surya Namaskar may be considered a mudra (Chapter 10) as it symbolically describes the cosmic wheel of life. In repeated practice the first and the thirteenth positions of the Surya Namaskar are identical, therefore the Surya Namaskar has twelve stages.

The symbolism and mantras of Surya Namaskar

Position 1   *Mantra* 'Om adi deva namah'
Here we face the spiritual sun. Standing upright with breath suspended, fully composed, we represent Purusha, the primeval god Adi Deva, at the very beginning of time.

Position 2   *Mantra* 'Om jata veda namah'
Having inspired and extended our arms back, we greet the dawn of a new universe. At this point knowledge is born, and the sum total of the Vedas—Jata Veda—is created like rays of light which necessarily illuminate one side of the universe throwing the other side into shadow.

Position 3   *Mantra* 'Om jyoti mey lingha namah'
Breathing out and bending forward with our hands on the ground, we represent the creation of the manifest universe of material. We represent the creative organ which built the universe of light—jyoti mey lingha—and consciousness enters into matter.

86

Position 4 *Mantra* 'Om divya svarupa namah'
Moving into a suitable position, yet keeping our attention on the Self represented by the sun, we are inspired to start the race which leads us deeper into
matter so that we may experience the universe of divine form—divya svarupa.

Position 5 *Mantra* 'Om anshu namah'
We form a bridge between the superior (anshu) levels and the inferior aspects
of the universe. We are midway in time and space between the whole universe
and the smallest particle (anshu) in the universe.

Position 6 *Mantra* 'Om rajaguna rupa namah'
Representing vibration, we are the embodiment of action—rajaguna rupa—and
play the role of the activist in the universe.

Position 7 *Mantra* 'Om Maha Vishnu namah'
Lying flat facing the earth, we breathe out to become totally involved in the
universe. Consciousness is fully invested in the material universe which it
maintains in its role as Maha Vishnu.

Position 8 *Mantra* 'Om amrit svarupa namah'
We cannot maintain the previous position for very long and must raise our
heads to glimpse the sun, representing the Self. Our inbreath represents the
inspiration we receive as we realise our life-giving immortal form—amrit
svarupa.

Position 9 *Mantra* 'Om ushra svarupa namah'
Filled with new life, we raise ourselves from the world of matter. Not quite free,
we form a bridge between absolute consciousness and chaotic unconsciousness.
This raising of consciousness comes to us all sooner or later just as the warming
sun—ushra svarupa—dawns each morning bringing the new day.

Position 10 *Mantra* 'Om hiran mey namah'
Fixing our consciousness on the Self, we lose no time in the race to perfection.
Only the pure gold—hiran mey—of the Self can survive the testing of life.

Position 11 *Mantra* 'Om akash vihari namah'
Our ego has totally expired as we submit absolutely, bowing before the Self.
Leaving our ego, we move in the void of space—akash vihari.

Position 12 *Mantra* 'Om adi teya namah'
Cosmically inspired, we welcome the Self as the prodigal son—adi
teya—returned.

Returning to the first position, we re-enter the ceaseless cosmic cycle of
involution and evolution.

9 Asanas

Asanas are performed in order to still the incessant activity of the body and personality. Asanas are not to be confused with athletic exercises, for while athletics is the science of action and movement, yoga is the science of stillness. A beginner usually finds it very difficult to even sit still, and he finds the stilling of mental and emotional activity yet more difficult. We are not still because our body and mind are full of tensions which, whether they originate in the physical body, the mind or elsewhere, are basically caused by breakdowns or blocks in communications. In the body, such a breakdown can be seen in the capillary restriction of blood flow to diseased areas, or it may be recognised as nervous tension and nervous inhibition. All these blocks are the results of unfulfilled needs which may be physiological, biological, psychological or parapsychological. Ultimately these needs arise from false identification, which is itself the product of suggestion and ultimately auto-suggestion.

Our psychosomatic tensions seem very real, but there is at least one stage magician who can take anyone from the audience and, by using a little hypnosis, can fold him up into a very tiny ball and put him into a ridiculously small box. The trick appears amazing, but it is a fairly well-known phenomenon in hypnosis. Great tensions may be produced in a person so that he cannot bend an arm, for example, or conversely the tensions in his body can be reduced to such an extent that he may be able to perform unusual feats.

Yogis learn from the whole of nature. In the past they observed that when we wake up in the mornings we stretch ourselves, as do animals although in different ways. In doing so we produce neuro-chemical effects which remove tensions from our body. The ancient yogis experimented and, from their discoveries about our body and mind, they devised a system of exercises which has come down to us as Hatha Yoga. They named the exercises after their functions, so the name of every asana is a formula telling us exactly what the posture does, not merely a label.

Let us examine some of the reasons for practising Hatha Yoga asanas. Most of the asanas are designed to work on a specific area of the body eg a chakra. Usually this is a special area of the spine or endocrine organ. Through certain kinds of bending and stretching, nerves may be turned on which have a tonic effect on muscles, visceral organs and the whole central nervous system. Specific bending and pressure can produce concentrations of blood flow to increase the production of endocrine hormones. Thus the main biological reason for practising asanas is to work on the endocrine system and the nervous system.

These systems work as an integrated unit and represent the directors of the body; thus by working on these, the entire body—consisting of muscles, bones, joints, circulatory system, alimentary system etc—benefits indirectly.

Through practising asanas the entire body may be rebuilt and brought to perfect health. The speed at which changes occur in the body depends upon the biological rhythms of the tissues concerned. For example, peptic ulcers may be healed in a fortnight and sugar diabetes can often be completely cured in about six weeks. Most of the hormonal problems, such as thyroid deficiency or excess, can be corrected in a few months, and whereas problems connected with the bones, such as arthritis, take up to a year or two to correct, certain aches and pains, including some headaches, can be cleared within seconds.

There are two major determinants of the length of time one should stay in a posture. In many postures you have to hold your breath in or out and so the length of time you can stay in the posture is limited to around thirty seconds or so. Certain postures, however, do not require the breath to be held, and normally you would maintain this posture long enough to allow the blood to circulate around your body once, that is about twenty-seven heart beats on average. Do not try to hold your postures for too long, for even if you do not make yourself ill, you are liable to retard your progress in mastering Hatha Yoga. In Hatha Yoga we work *with* our body and not against it, doing everything easily and gently. Breath is sometimes held in and sometimes held out according to the kind of effects that are required, the most important being the electromagnetic and pranic effects.

As has already been discussed, the body consists of a number of centres (chakras) which are analogous to transistors in electronics, and these are connected by countless conducting pathways called nadis in yoga. We may put these pathways and centres together in different arrangements to produce different effects, rather like having a do-it-yourself electronics kit with which it is possible to create either a record player, a radio, a television or a negative ion generator, according to the way we put the connections and transistors together.

Finally, the most important aspect of the asana is the concentration. 90 per cent of all yoga practice is concentration and without proper concentration the postures are merely external replicas of the asanas. By concentration we can easily increase the circulation in any part of the body and thus counteract reduced circulation produced by psychosomatic tension. Through concentration we are able to direct plasma, ionised gases and liquids in our body, and we can also direct our pranas to produce healing, growth and expansion.

As you become more advanced in asanas you will be able to include the practice of Mantra in your postures. These, of course, will be silent and are practised in order to direct and control mental waves in order to maximise the effects.

In practising Hatha Yoga it must be clearly understood that the body has its own intelligence, otherwise you are liable to do yourself an injury. If you practice the technique properly you cannot go wrong, but the body has inbuilt defences to prevent you from attempting anything you should not practise. If you cannot perform an asana using the proper technique, do not force your body or use any tricks to get into the posture. Do not attempt a posture too many times; twice in any one session is plenty. Practise all postures carefully and cleanly. Regardless of your original physical condition, by observing the proper techniques and practising regularly and effectively under a good teacher you should master all the postures within two or three years.

Some asanas bring great pressure to bear on certain parts of the body, the neck region for example, and so it is important to perform complementary asanas one after another to balance the pressures.

The Order of an Asana Programme

The order in which you practise an asana programme is most important as the production of one hormone may well trigger the production of another in a different gland. Thus postures executed in different orders have different effects. There is a general rule, however, which requires that those asanas which effect the highest centres in the body—the pineal, pituitary and thyroid, rather than the adrenals, gonads and pancreas—should be practised first.

It must be realised that some hormones are desirable for yoga states while others are not, and by designing your asana programme so that you start working on the higher centres you can select out the hormones you want, and need, to produce. Research has shown that it is quite possible to be very specific both in the production of hormones and in the training of other so-called 'autonomic' functions in the body. Thus the first asana to be practised in an established yoga asana session is the Sirshasana, which works on the brain, the pineal and pituitary glands. [Note: this is a very powerful posture and should not be practised until at least a year of really efficient Hatha Yoga work under a good teacher has been carried out. Even this may be far too soon for most people.] After working on the head and its glands, attention must then be turned to the organs in the neck, such as the thyroid and parathyroids. Asanas such as the Sarvangasana and the Matsyasana would therefore come next. In this way you would work through an asana programme, finishing with postures such as the Garudasana which works on the gonads.

Imposed upon these considerations is another system of ordering which should be followed in designing a programme. It can be summarised thus:

Headstand
Forward bending
Backward bending
Twisting
Further forward bending
Further backward bending
Standing bending
Standing balances

90

Complex exercises
Mudras
Bandhas
Kriyas

A brief look at this list will show that the forward and backward bending exercises balance each other up and prepare for the twisting exercises. These first three groups of exercises are performed on the floor followed by the standing bending exercises and the balances. At first you will find the balances are much more difficult to do at this point in the programme but they are far more significant at this stage. Having worked up all kinds of energies and moved your pranas around your body during the bending and twisting, you then have to balance them up. Complex exercises are a small group of combined exercises which do not clearly fall into the previous categories. Mudras, bandhas and kriyas are rather more advanced exercises than the asanas and they are practised after the body and mind have been prepared by the rest of the programme. When you begin practice of yoga asanas under a teacher, you will find that some of the postures are much easier for you than others. If you are in a class with other students, you may discover that your fellow students can perform better than you on some postures and not as well on others. In other words the different psychosomatic tensions within every individual will show up in their different abilities to perform the postures. In fact, it is quite easy to predict where you will experience stiffness according to your personality.

The relation of psychosomatic tensions to personality is a most interesting subject, on which we do not have room to elaborate here. It is essential knowledge for yoga teachers but is not essential for students initially. However, do make sure you have a good teacher as he or she will be able to answer all your questions on these matters. You may also find that one side of your body is freer and less tense than the other. This is caused by the left/right differences in the body, particularly in the brain, but this imbalance will work out with practice.

After an asana programme you should feel refreshed and full of energy. If you feel exhausted or tired then you have not been practising yoga but have been doing something which you think is yoga but it is in fact athletics. Yoga practices conserve energy and build up strength rather than expend vast amounts of energy as do athletic practices.

Special note

It is of utmost importance to find yourself a good teacher. If you attempt to teach yourself yoga you are likely to become ill. The major mistake made by students is to try to practise either too many or too advanced postures before they are able. They are keen but foolish. The problem of students trying to short-cut proper yoga practice is not a new one, there has always been a science of yoga medicine for students who are suffering from illnesses caused by mal-practice. The Shatkarmasangraha is devoted entirely to such problems and the

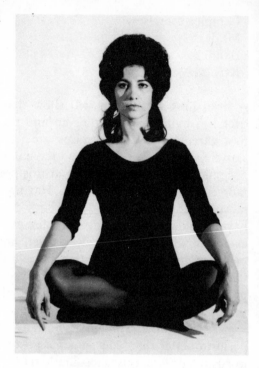

fifth chapter of the *Hathapradipika* is concerned with suitable cures. Yoga asanas, when done properly, are powerful, efficient, effective exercises which have definite, predictable, positive results. When they are done incorrectly they will either have an entirely neutral effect and produce no results at all or else prove extremely detrimental.

The following Asana methods have been selected as a representative cross-section.

Sukhasana

Sukhasana means the 'easy posture' and the method is very simple. Sit cross-legged on the ground with the back straight and upright and your hands one on top of each other in your lap with your palms upwards, or alternatively rest your wrists on your knees.

Beginners should have little difficulty with this posture as most people can sit in this position from the first. It is the usual posture for practising Pranayama and for achieving composure before starting a yoga asana programme.

Vajrasana

Vajra is sometimes translated as 'a thunderbolt' which is known to be the weapon of Indra, one of the chief gods of Hindu mythology, who is the executive of the indriyas—the senses. *Vajra* comes from the word *va* which means 'to go' or 'to move' and *ra* as in Radiant', 'radiate' energy. Vajra then, is the posture which assists the collection of the psychic energy which is dispersed throughout

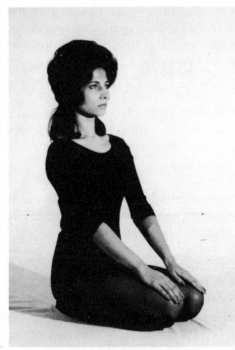

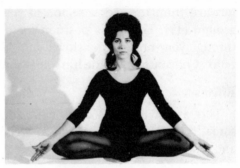

16 Badrasana stage 1

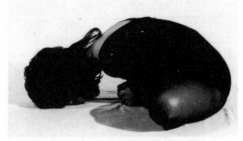

15 Vajrasana   17 Badrasana stage 2

the body and sublimates it for use in concentration and meditative work. The vajra is also the name given to one of the nadis within the Sushumna.

Method

Kneel down with your knees and heels together, Sit back on your heels, keeping your back upright and your head slightly down to keep your back straight (15). Place your hands on your thighs and gently relax.

Effects

This again is an excellent posture for attentive work. It restricts blood flow to the legs, directing it up into the trunk to nourish the internal organs. It is an excellent position in which to practise various eye and neck exercises.

The Bhadrasana

Bhadra is usually translated as 'auspicious', 'prosperous', or even 'happy'. This asana has been given this name because it releases hormonal energies which enhance the appearance of the practiser.

Method

Sit on the ground with your back straight and legs extended together in front of you. Bring your heels and soles of your feet together and pull them towards your body (16). Gently press your knees down to the ground with extended arms, breathing normally. Breathe in, and then breathe out as you bend forward from the sacral region of your spine and touch your forehead on the ground (17). Hold this position for a few seconds, then gradually breathe in through your nose as you slowly sit up. Remove your legs from this position and relax. Concentrate on the hip joints throughout this exercise.

Effects

This asana removes calcification from the hip joints and relieves psycho-somatic tensions in the sacral and coccygeal regions and in the thighs, knees and ankles.

Siddhasana

Siddha means 'attainment' and a siddha is someone who has made progress in yoga and attained a certain degree of self-mastery and harmony of personality. In the *Hathapradipika* it says that the siddhas believe that just as temperance (mitahana) is the most important of the yamas and harmlessness or non-violence (Ahimsa) is foremost among the niyamas, so Siddhasana is the most important of the asanas (while Ahimsa is normally listed as a yama, when it becomes a positive practice rather than a restraint it is a niyama). Of the eighty-four asanas, Siddhasana should be practised daily as it purifies the 72,000 nadis. The word nadi is used here for a channel for transmission of food or drink, blood or air and nervous impulse or energy of some kind. The yogi who contemplates atman, observes temperance and practices Siddhasana for twelve years attains the yoga siddhis.

The Siddhasana is an excellent posture for adopting the three bandhas, which are described elsewhere in the book.

Method

Sit on the floor with your legs stretched straight in front of you. Bend the left leg at the knee and, taking hold of the left foot with your hands, place the heel near the perineum and rest the sole of the left foot against the right thigh. Bend the right leg at the knee and place the right foot over the left ankle, keeping the right heel against the pubic bone and with the sole of the right foot between the thigh and the calf of the left leg. Do not rest your body on your heel. There are a number of positions for your arms but the traditional posture is to have your arms stretched out in front of you with the backs of your hands resting on your knees so that your palms face upwards. Place your hands in the Jnana Mudra (18).

This position may be repeated with the legs in the opposite order, that is with your right heel near the perineum and the left foot over the right ankle. This posture is particularly good for practising such techniques as Tratakam and Drishti, which are described later.

Effects

There is a general reduction of blood flow to the legs so that blood is redirected up into the trunk of the body, benefitting the lumbar region and the

94

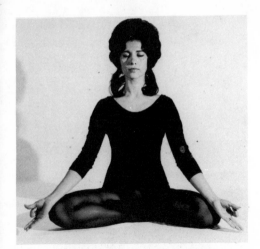

18 Siddhasana

abdomen particularly. It tones the lower region of the spine and the abdominal organs. This asana also reduces stiffness in the knees and ankles. The Siddhasana is particularly good for achieving an alert attentive state of mind for practice of concentration.

Padmasana

Padma is sometimes translated as 'lotus' and so the posture is known as the lotus seat, or lotus position. *Pad* means 'foot' and *Ma* comes from a word meaning 'authority' or 'knowledge'. Padmasana can thus be thought of as being the seat which brings one to the base of knowledge. Teachers say that just to sit in the lotus posture is a reminder to the aspiring yogi to be like the lotus plant, with its roots in the soil or matter and its face pointing upwards towards heaven.

Method

Sit on the ground with your legs stretched out in front of you and slightly apart, and your back straight. Take your right foot and place it high on the left thigh with the sole of the foot turned up; rest your right knee on the ground. Then take your left foot and place it high on the right thigh with the sole facing up and the left knee resting on the ground. Your feet should press into the soft pressure points at the top of your groin (19). Breathe naturally and concentrate on balance and harmony. Repeat the same posture, either later in the programme or when you next practise, with the left foot placed first on the right thigh and the right foot placed above the left thigh. It is essential to have the spine upright and straight with the chin slightly down so that the cervical region is in a proper line with the rest of the spine.

Effect

This asana provides a firm position such as is required for the practice of Pranayama or meditation. Again the flow of blood to the legs is constricted and redirected to the internal organs.

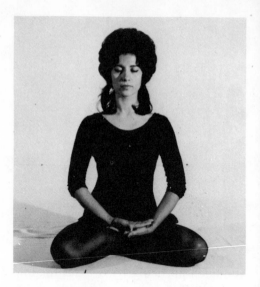

19 Padmasana

This posture is symbolic of the law of trinity eg God the Father, God the Son and God the Holy Ghost; Brahma, Vishnu and Shiva in Hinduism; Sattvaguna, Rajoguna, Tamoguna in Yoga Samkhya philosophy; thesis, antithesis and synthesis in western philosophy. The Padmasana is the basis of several other postures.

Sirshasana

Sirsh means 'the head' and the Sirshasana, also called the King of Asanas, is one of the most important of all the postures. Normally it should not be attempted until the student has practised effective yoga for at least one complete year as there can be many hidden dangers in Sirshasana. Your teacher will tell you when you are ready to start practising this posture. Also the Sirshasana should not be undertaken immediately after any strenuous exercise; at least half an hour should elapse. Ideally Sirshasana should start your asana programme.

Method

Kneel on your mat and rest your forearms on the ground with your elbows shoulder width apart. Interlock your fingers. Rest the crown of your head on your mat so that the back of your head touches your hands. Raise your knees from the ground bringing your toes nearer to your head and when your back is more or less vertical, gradually raise your knees taking your feet off the ground. Straighten your spine and head and finally raise your legs to the vertical position (20). Balance with your body extended straight, legs together.

Breathe gently relaxing in the Sirshasana. Apart from a slight pressure on the top of your crown, your body should experience no strain or tensions. Maintain this posture for about one minute at first and extend this time under the instruction of your teacher. Concentrate on the top of your head.

Gently lower your feet and legs to the ground, taking the weight on your toes

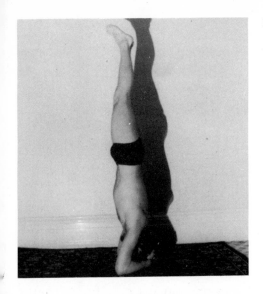

and then on your knees. Sit in the Vajrasana and gently pass your hands over your face and down to your legs. Relax for a few seconds before continuing.

Effects

This asana works on the Sahasaram, stimulating the pineal and the pituitary glands and thus benefitting the entire body and personality. It tones up particularly the nervous, digestive and endocrine systems. Under special instruction neurasthania, dyspepsia, congested liver and spleen, visceratosis, hernia and certain types of asthma can be effectively treated with Sirshasana. Last but not least, it keeps you youthful and vigorous by counteracting the ageing effects of gravity.

Note: People suffering from the following disorders should not attempt the Sirshasana: aching or running ears, weak eye capillaries, very high or very low blood pressure, weak heart, chronic nasal catarrh and chronic constipation.

Sarvangasana

Sarvangasana comes from *Sarva* meaning 'everything' or 'the whole' and *anga* meaning a 'limb' or 'body'. The Sarvangasana effects and benefits the entire body.

Method

Lie flat on your back with your arms by your side and palms downwards. Keep your legs extended together and your knees straight. Breathe in through your nose and hold your breath as you slowly raise your legs, keeping them straight throughout. Allow your trunk to come up, and support your back with your hands. Keeping your elbows on the ground, straighten up to the vertical position with your body absolutely straight from your shoulders, your head and neck at right angles to your body, and your chin pressed hard into your chest forming

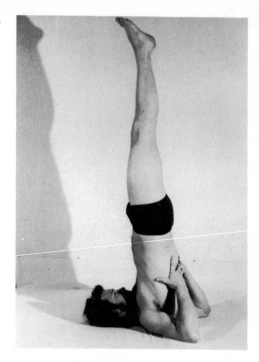

the chin lock (21). Breathe normally and easily in the pose and concentrate on the base of your throat. Hold this position for about thirty seconds at first. Breathe in and then hold your breath as you slowly move your legs back and over your head to a balanced position; then remove your hands and place them by the sides of your body. Slowly bring your legs and trunk down, keeping your legs absolutely straight to avoid any possible jolting of the base of your spine; do not bang your heels down. Relax flat on the ground, breathing out.

It is very important to keep your legs straight at all times; many students are tempted to bend their knees but this will alter the position of the spine. Do not point your toes but keep your feet relaxed, otherwise you may well get cramp. If you find it impossible to get up into the Sarvangasana using the proper technique it simply means that your body is not ready, so do not force it.

Effects

This asana awakens the Vishuddhi Chakra. It is a unique pose as, being an inverse position, it tends to counteract the ageing effects of gravity and rejuvenate the whole system. This posture improves the functional activities of the thyroid and parathyroid by increasing blood supply to this organ through the superior thyroid artery. The Sarvangasana has a beneficial effect on the sex glands of both sexes, arresting age degeneration. It also relieves gastro-intestinal disorders, dispepsia, constipation, displaced uterus, hernia and varicose veins.

Note: This posture should always be followed by its complementary, the Matsyasana, as there is a certain amount of residual strain in the neck muscles which must be balanced by the neck being pressed in the opposite direction. If the two

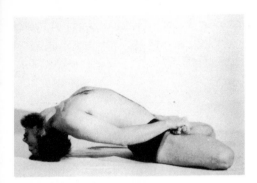

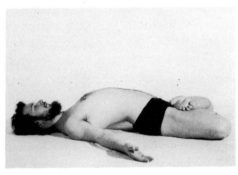

23   Matsyasana rest position

are not performed in conjunction it is very likely that you will suffer from head-aches or other problems. These headaches may come immediately or may be de-layed for several hours or even until the next day. Over an extended period, a shorter period if you are older and not in such good physical condition, you will sustain neck damage unless you practise this asana properly and balance it up with its complementary.

Matsyasana

Matsya is usually translated as 'fish', but it comes from a root word *mat* which means something like 'lively'. The Matsyasana enlivens the metabolism of the body.

Method

Sit on the ground in the Padmasana. Breathe in through the nose and hold your breath as you carefully lean back onto your elbows. Arch your back and, keep-ing your folded legs flat on the ground, turn your head back and gently rest your weight on the top of your head. Bring your arms forward and hold your toes (22). Breathe normally in this position for about fifteen seconds, concentrating on the back of the neck. Place your elbows on the ground once more and put your hands under your thighs. Using your arms as levers, ease yourself gently on to your shoulders. Hold your breath in as you do this. Place your neck and the back of your head flat on the ground, retaining an arch like a tunnel underneath the small of the back and keeping your folded legs flat on the ground (23). Rest in this position for a few seconds and then place your hands one on top of the other, palms down, underneath the small of your back; breathe in and hold your breath. Press gently on the ground with your hands and you will find that you can sit up very easily. Take your legs out of the Padmasana and relax, breathing normally.

Effects

This asana works on the Vishuddhi Chakra. It can help the thyroid and parathyroid glands, tone up the pituitary and pineal glands, benefit the neck and chest, and arrest sexual and abdominal degeneration. From above this posture suggests the shape of a fish, and it is interesting that you can float in water in this position for long periods. The spine is benefitted particularly in the cervical area and also in the sacral region during the rest position. With the left hand holding the right foot, and the right hand holding the left foot, the electrical and magnetic currents of the body are balanced. The Matsyasana is normally used to complement the Sarvangasana.

Gomukhasana

Gomukh is usually translated as 'the head of a cow', based on the idea that *go* means 'cow', but in the Vedas the word *go* is used to mean 'light' in the sense of 'light of consciousness', and it is this word which appears in Gomukh and also in Gomamsa. *Gomukh* means 'light in or of the head', and the effect of the Gomukhasana is to wake up the brain. After practice of the Gomukhasana you will indeed feel somewhat light-headed.

Method

Sit in the Vajrasana. Raise your right arm and bend your forearm down behind your back with your right elbow pointing upwards. Take your left arm behind your back and bend your arm so that your left elbow points downwards and you can hold your right hand by clasping the fingers (24). Close your eyes and breathe in through your nose as you slowly lower your trunk and head to the ground, keeping your back as straight as you can and your bottom touching your heels. Rest your forehead on the ground in front of you and hold your breath in this position, for about thirty seconds at first, concentrating on the centre of your forehead (25). Now slowly raise your head and trunk, blowing your cheeks out as you breathe out through your mouth. Sit up and unclasp your hands. Repeat this exercise with your left elbow uppermost.

Effects

This asana helps awaken the Ajna Chakra. It works on the shoulder joints to remove and prevent further calcification. Having the legs folded under the body in this manner helps the flow of blood to the trunk and to the brain. The extra blood supply to the head deeply nourishes the complexion and removes wrinkles, while the pituitary and the pineal glands are also benefitted, thus helping the general body health. Bloodflow is restricted to the lower arm in this posture

100

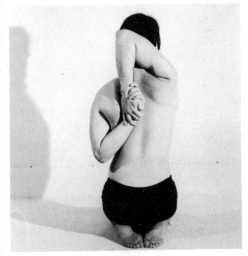

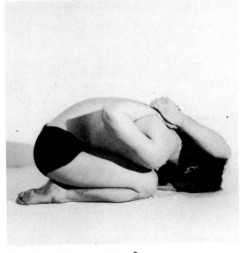

24 Gomukhasana stage 1   25 Gomukhasana stage 2

and correspondingly increased through the appropriate carotid artery to magnetise that side of the brain.

Paschimotanasana

Paschima literally means 'the west'. In yoga, the back is considered to be towards the west and the front is towards the east; hence we always face the east. The head or top end of the body is considered to be the north aand the feet are considered to be towards the south. *Utana* means 'to stretch', and thus Paschimotanasana is the posture which stretches the west part of the body.

Method

Lie flat on your back with your arms by your sides and your legs extended together. Breathe in through your nose as you raise your arms back over your head. Hold your breath and sit up slowly, moving from your hips and keeping your arms, body and trunk in line. Place your chest on your thighs, and your chin and forehead on your shins, breathing out as you do so. Hold your position with your breath out. Concentrate on the sacral portion of your spine, keep your legs absolutely straight and take hold of your toes, placing your elbows on the ground (26). Hold this position for as long as is comfortable (about twenty seconds at first) and then slowly breathe in through your nose as you sit up.

Effects

This exercise works on the Svadisthana Chakra. It benefits the spine, particularly the sacral region, removing psychosomatic tensions from that area. It strengthens the abdomen and loosens the hamstrings in the back of the legs. There is a gentle stomach massage in this posture which aids digestion and helps to get rid of constipation.

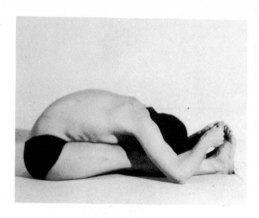

Janusirasana

Ja means 'born, offspring', *nu* means 'now, still, even' and *sir* 'the seat of consciousness'. Janusir then refers to the process of being reborn in consciousness.

Method

Sit on the floor with the legs straight and slightly apart and the back upright. Place your right foot on your left groin with the sole uppermost and keep the right knee flat on the ground. Breathe in through your nose and, keeping your back straight, lean forward from the hips and clasp your left heel with both hands. Place your head on your left shin, hold your breath in and concentrate on your left kidney (27). Hold this position for as long as is comfortable—about fifteen or twenty seconds initially. Breathe out through the nose as you slowly sit up and relax. Repeat this exercise but reversing the right and left leg positions.

Effects

In performing this asana the Svadisthana Chakra is awakened. This exercise stretches the hamstrings of the legs and works particularly on the sacral area of the spine. It also benefits the kidneys, the adrenals and the abdominal organs in general. The kidneys are very difficult organs to get near and this exercise is one of the few postures which works fairly directly upon them. Notice that the breathing here is the reversal of the normal yoga procedure; normally we breathe out as we go forward and breathe in as we come up. In this posture, however, we breathe in as we go forward in order to flatten the diaphragm and thus push the abdominal organs beneath it down and forward. The heel should be placed high up on the groin of the opposite leg in such a position that it goes underneath the rib cage as you bend forward. The combined effect of bending forward, bringing the heel up underneath the rib cage and holding the breath in so that the abdominal organs are lowered is to bring the kidney into a position where they may be gently massaged by other tissues through the heel.

In yoga we know that when the sole of the foot is in close proximity to the kidneys a bio-energetic (pranic) feed-back circuit is established which steps up nervous energies enabling the practitioner to be 'reborn in consciousness'.

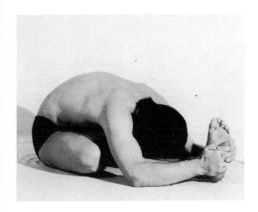

Bandha Janusir

Bandha means 'control' and by modifying the simple Janusirasana your bio-energy may be controlled a little more precisely.

Method

Practise the Janusirasana as described above. When your right foot is resting on your left thigh, take your right hand behind your back and hold your right toes from the left side (28). Repeat the other side.

Effects

This produces all the advantages of the Janusirasana but with additional bio-energetic effects. Additionally, the blood flow to the right arm, which is held behind the back, is restricted. There will tend to be increased blood supply to that side of the brain through the cartoid artery. This will charge the appropriate hemisphere with Prana and magnify the functioning of this part of the brain.

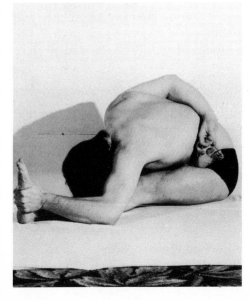

28   Bandha Janusir

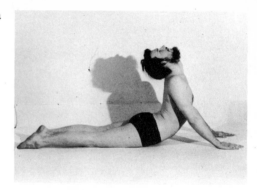

Bhujangasana

Bhuj means 'bend' or 'curve', *ga* means 'going' or 'moving in' and thus bhujanga means moving in curves or in a wave-like motion, as a serpent does. Proper practice of the Bhujangasana will make the whole body vibrate during the relaxation period after the posture, as the Kundalini energies—represented by a coiled snake—will rise and invigorate the nervous system.

Method

Lie flat on your front with your forehead on the ground and legs and feet together. Place your hands, palms downwards, under your shoulders and slightly in front of them, with your fingers pointing forward. Keep your elbows into your sides. Breathe in and slowly raise your head, then push your body up by straightening your arms and bending from the waist; relax your bottom and legs completely. Look back over your body, making sure that your pelvis and legs remain flat on the ground, and hold your breath (29). Hold this position for about fifteen or twenty seconds whilst concentrating on the small of your back. Breathe out gently through your nose as you first bring your head back into line with your trunk, and then lower your shoulders and the rest of your body to the ground by bending and relaxing your arms. Relax in the horizontal position and breathe normally.

Effects

This pose works on the Manipura Chakra. It benefits the back and abdominal muscles, corrects displacement tendencies in the spinal column and works particularly on the lumbar region. It also has beneficial effects on the spinal column, the parasympathetic and the sympathetic nervous systems, and can also alleviate indigestion and flatulence. This posture should normally be followed by the Salabasana which acts as a complementary to it.

Salabhasana

Sa means 'sharpen' or 'sharp' and *labh* means 'to obtain' or 'to catch sight of, perceive, ascertain'. The Salabhasana is thus the technique which sharpens up your perception.

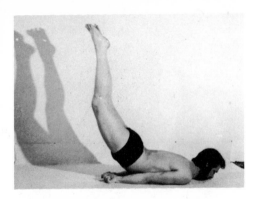

30 Salabhasana stage 1

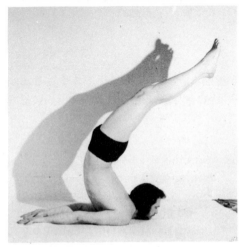

31 Salabhasana stage 2

Method

Lie flat on your front with your legs extended together and your feet flat. Lay your forehead on the ground and your arms by your sides. Clench your fists and place them under your pelvis, keeping your arms fully extended. Breathe in through your nose and hold your breath as you raise your legs with a fairly quick motion (this is unusual in yoga). Keep your legs absolutely straight and, without bending the knees, hold this position for about ten to fifteen seconds (30); concentrate on the small of your back. Still holding your breath, slowly lower your legs to the ground and then relax, breathing out.

Effects

Like its complementary, the Bhujangasana, this asana works on the Manipura Chakra. The posture benefits the pelvis and abdomen, strengthens the back muscles and aids circulation in the legs. The Bhujangasana works on the part of the body above the small of the back while the Salabhasana works on the remainder, particularly the lower part of the back. However, as the Salabhasana improves with practice, the technique changes a little (31) and it becomes more or less the reverse of the Sarvangasana or the Halasana.

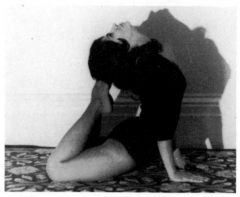

32 Bhujangendrasana

Bhujangendra

Bhujang was defined in Bhujangasana and *endra* is 'mental power'; hence Bhujangendra is the practice whereby mental power can be stepped up and Kundalini may be turned on.

Method

Lie flat on the floor on your stomach. Bend your elbows and place the palms on the floor on either side of your waist. Breathe in and lift your head and trunk, stretching the arms fully. The weight of the body should be felt mainly in the pelvic region and on the thighs. Raise your feet and place your head on the soles of your feet (32). Hold your breath, concentrating on the small of your back. Hold the position for about fifteen or twenty seconds at first and then gently relax, lowering your feet and legs, bend your elbows and relax the front of your body, first lowering your head and then your trunk. Breathe out and relax flat.

Effects

This asana works on the Manipura Chakra. The abdominal organs are massaged and all the glands, particularly the thyroid, parathyroid, adrenals and gonads, receive a rich supply of blood. Psychosomatic tensions are removed from the small of the back, the lumbar and sacral regions, the pelvis and the front of the legs.

Dhanurasana

Dha means 'placing' or 'putting, bestowing' and *nur* has the double meaning being 'still, now' and also having the idea of sound, such as the aum. In the *Hathapradipika,* it says: 'Internal sound (nada) is a snare for catching the inner deer. It is the hunter that can kill the captured deer (the mind)'. Again it says: 'The whole mind standing still like the deer that is attracted by the sound of the bells is easily killed provided the archer is skillful in aiming the arrow'. The aim of the Dhanurasana is to gain control over the metabolic processes, ie still the constant mental and physical changes within the body.

106

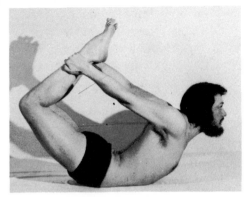
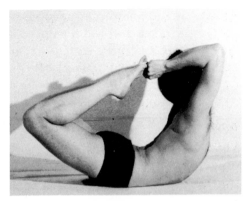

33 Dhanurasana method one   34 Dhanurasana method two

Method one

Lie flat on your front with your arms by your sides; have your palms upwards and your legs together. Bend your knees and bring your feet up carefully. Grasp both your ankles simultaneously and, holding your ankles, lie with your forehead on the ground for a few moments. Breathe in and hold your breath as you pull your body up into the Dhanur position (33). Only your navel area should now be touching the ground. Hold your head back as far as you can, looking over your head, and keep your knees and feet together. Hold your breath in this position for only ten or fifteen seconds initially and concentrate on the small of your back. Still holding your breath, gently lower your body to the ground and relax, breathing out before you let go of your ankles. The technique used to come out of this posture is very important because if the breath is not retained pressures on the diaphragm will be unbalanced and if the feet are released before breathing out and relaxing, there will be residual tension in the back, and in this condition it is very easy to pull a small muscle through imbalance. The complementary Uttitha Kummerasana should be practised after the Dhanurasana.

Effects

This exercise awakens the Manipura Chakra. It stretches the muscles of the abdomen and hips and massages the back muscles. It also corrects spinal curvature tendencies and reduces abdominal fat. This posture alleviates stomach gas conditions and invigorates the appetite. Psychosomatic tensions are removed from lumbar region and from the fronts of the legs and hamstrings which are innervated by lumbar nerves.

Method two

Lie flat on your stomach with your arms by your sides, palms down. Let your legs part a little and bend your knees, bringing your feet up. Rotate your hands outwards so that your palms face upwards. Grasp your big toes between your first and second fingers. Breathe in and hold your breath as you rotate your elbows out and above your body as you pull your body into the bow-like asana. Bring your knees and feet together (34). Hold the position with your breath retained for about fifteen seconds. Concentrate on the small of the back. Relax your legs and let them part slightly as you rotate your elbows back to their previous position, and then lower your knees to the ground. Breathe gently, and carefully let go of your feet. Relax.

Effects

This is an intensified version of the technique described above. Its effects are similar but new work is carried out on the shoulders which must become very supple.

Halasana

The word *hal* in Sanskrit is composed of two letters *ha* and *la*. *Ha* comes from a root word meaning 'to leave kill or quit' and *la* comes from a word meaning 'pertaining to physical or sexual behaviour'. Thus the Halasana is indeed one of the first asanas in which most students discover they can feel really comfortable and are able to transcend their bodily feelings. Usually *hal* is simply translated as 'the plough'. The Halasana ploughs back psycho-sexual energy, otherwise fruitlessly scattered, and makes it available for higher mental work.

Method

Lie flat on your back with your arms by your sides, palms down. Keep your feet together as you breathe in and, holding your breath, slowly raise your legs, keeping them absolutely straight. Bring your legs back over your head and slowly breathe out as your legs are lowered until your toes touch the ground. Now hold your breath in as you take your feet back as far as they will go behind your head until your chin is pressing hard into your chest (35). You will feel the centre of gravity of your body near the middle of your head. Keep your feet at right angles to your legs and hold this posture for about thirty seconds breathing normally but shallowly, as the throat and chest are rather constricted in this position, and concentrating on the base of your throat. Then bring your feet back a little towards your head so that your back comes down slightly, breathe in and hold your breath as you raise your legs back over your head and then slowly lower first your back to the ground and then your legs, still keeping them absolutely straight. Relax flat on the ground, breathing gently.

Effects

This is another asana which awakens the Vishuddhi Chakra, and also stimulates the Anhata Chakra. This exercise alleviates diseases of the joints and reduces abdominal and chest fat. It strengthens the abdominal and back muscles, relieves back ache doing special work on the thoracic region, and renders the spine very elastic. It improves the upright standing posture and stimulates the thyroid and parathyroid glands to the benefit of the entire body. In this position

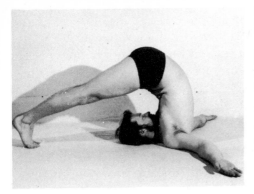 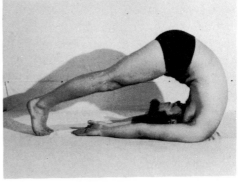

35 Halasana method one   36 Halasana method two

pressure is placed upon the carotid sinuses at the sides of the neck and the heart rate and blood pressure tend to be reduced. This posture should be followed by the Suptravajrasana, which balances up the pressures on the neck region.

Method two

In this version follow exactly the same technique as outlined above. However, whilst you are in the posture, extend your arms and bring them along the ground to place them together above your head (36). Hold this position in exactly the same way as above, but return your arms to the first position before coming out of the posture.

Effects

The same as those described above but this technique tends to improve the bend a little higher in the cervical region of the spine.

Suptavajrasana

Supta means 'sleep', and the Suptavajrasana is the posture through which the sensory energy may be overcome, mastered and conserved.

Method

Sit in the Vajrasana, breathe in and hold your breath as you lean back onto your elbows. Arch your back and rest your weight on the top of your head; place the palms of your hand together with fingers pointing up and gently squeeze your sides with your elbows (37). Breathe gently in this position and hold it for about thirty seconds initially. Keep your knees flat on the ground and concentrate on the base of your neck. Breathe in, hold your breath, and, using your arms as levers, gently lower yourself to the ground so that the back of your head and shoulders are flat on the ground (38). With your hands and arms relaxed by your sides, breathe gently for about fifteen seconds and concentrate on the sacral region of your spine. Place your hands one on top of the other, palms down, underneath the small of your back, breathe in and gently push yourself up into the Vajrasana. Relax and breathe normally.

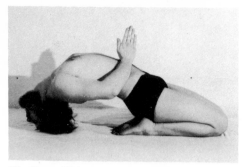

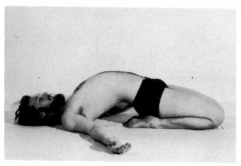

37 Supta Vajrasana

38 Supta Vajrasana rest position

Effects

This posture works on both the Vishuddhi and Svadisthana Chakras. It benefits the spine, especially the sacral, lumbar and cervical regions, relieves aching and tired legs, recharges the pelvic energies and rejuvenates the sexual apparatus.

Eka Pada Rajakapotasana

Eka means 'one', *pada* means 'foot' and this is the one-footed version of the Rajakapotasana. *Raja* indicates the 'highest' or 'supreme', *ka* refers to the Self and *pota* means 'youth, child'. The Rajakapotasana is an exercise which has the effect of producing the supreme childlike qualities of youth and non-agression, peace. Kapota is the name for a pigeon or dove which symbolises these qualities by its manner. The dove represents the positive Anhata Chakra qualities, with its wings analogous to the lungs and its body likened to the heart.

Method

Sit on the floor with your legs stretched out in front of you. Bend the right knee and, keeping it on the ground, place the right foot so that the right heel touches the left groin. Stretch the left leg back so that the front of the left thigh, the knee, shin and instep touch the floor. Bend your head back with your chest protruding and first with your left, and then your right hands catch hold of your left foot and rest your head on the sole (39). Stay in the pose for about ten seconds, breathing gently concentrating on the centre of your chest. Repeat with the other leg.

Effects

The blood circulation in the lower region of the spine is improved, the neck and shoulder muscles are exercised, and the thyroids, parathyroids, thymus, adrenals and gonads are stimulated. This asana works predominantly on the Svadisthana and the Anahata Chakras.

Chakrasana

The word *chakra* means 'a wheel, centre, circle or nodal point'. The Chakrasana is a complete technique for stimulating all the Chakras.

110

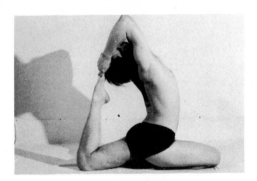

Method

Lie flat on your back with your feet drawn up to your buttocks, keeping your legs together. Revolve your hands backwards in a circular motion so that your elbows are uppermost and the palms of your hands are flat on the ground by the sides of your head, pointing towards your body. Breathe in, hold your breath, and slowly push your body up, raising your navel to the highest point (40). Concentrate on the small of your back whilst you breathe gently and hold this posture for about thirty seconds. Breathe in and hold your breath as you gently lower your body to the ground and relax.

Effects

This asana produces complete spinal stimulation and spinal correction. It benefits the reproductive system, helps to correct constipation and digestive troubles and tends to prevent excess weight and tones up the whole body. It stimulates all the Chakras.

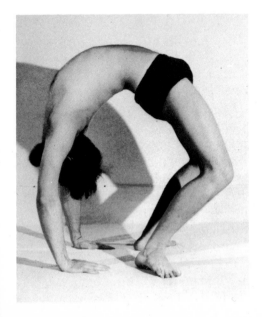

40   Chakrasana

Ushtrasana

Ush means 'the warming light of dawn'. When we perceive an answer to a problem we say that 'light has been thrown on the problem'. Our intellect, which is
associated with the Manipura Chakra, may work until a solution 'dawns' upon
us. The Ushtrasana stimulates the Manipura Chakra to brighten our intellect.
A good intellect may be used to analyse our experience of the universe to protect
us from illusion. *Ushtra* means 'that which protects us from ignorance and
stimulates our mind to throw light on previously dim areas of knowledge'. For
those who thirst for knowledge and hunger for spiritual food, the Ushtrasana
can release a store of knowledge unsuspected in a barren environment. Thus the
camel can survive in a desert by tapping its store of nourishment in its hump-
also called *ushtra*.

Method

Sit upright on your knees. Breathe in and hold your breath as you lean back
slowly and, keeping your arms straight, take hold of your heels. With your arms
still straight, bend your head back, looking over your head. Press your pelvis
forward, hollowing your back (41). Breathe shallowly and gently in this position, concentrating on the small of your back for about fifteen seconds. Breathe
in and hold your breath as you straighten up, letting go of your heels. Relax,
breathing gently.

Effects

This pose benefits the lumbar area of the spine, aids the neck, discourages
stomach fat and benefits the reproductive organs. It awakens the Manipura
Chakra.

Matsyendra

The yoga story runs that Lord Shiva was talking to his wife Parvati, explaining
Hatha Yoga postures to her, when a fish nearby in the water spoke up saying,
'Yes, I have heard all that before, but it is of no use to me because I am a fish'.
Parvati took pity on this fish and transformed it into a human being. It so happened that the fish was turned into a human being just as Shiva was explaining a
twisting posture and thus the posture became known as Matsyendra. Another
story tells how Matsyendra, a fish, swimming past a hermitage where he overheard a sage complaining that he was getting old and no longer had the health
of youth to help him continue his studies which were so important. Matsyendra
struck a bargain with this sage, saying that he would teach him a method by
which he would regain his youth, if in return the sage would transform him into
a man. Matsyendra taught the sage the twisting posture which is now labelled
Matsyendrasana. In fact Matsyendra was a great yogi and the founder of the in-
fluential Nath school of yoga.

We have already seen that *Matsya* means 'the power of enlivening, of inner-
vating, of turning on the energies' of the body and mind, and that *endra* refers

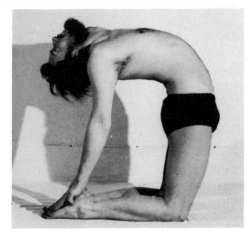

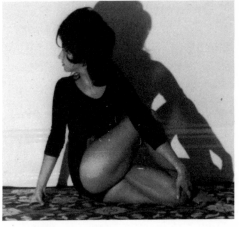

41 Ushtrasana   42 Matsyendrasana

to mental powers. Matsyendrasana is then one of the greatest of all the traditional yoga postures, having the effect of enlivening the brain and the entire body to raise mental alertness and give great bodily health.

Method

Sit on the ground with your legs stretched out in front of you; bend your right knee and place the right foot high on the left groin, take the left foot and lift it over the right thigh, placing it on the ground by the outside of the right knee. Breathe gently and turn to your extreme left. Bring the right shoulder over the left knee and hold the right foot with the right hand. Turn your neck and head as far as you can to your left and take the left arm behind the back to hold the left ankle with the left hand (42). Breathing during this posture should be fairly shallow and will be slightly faster because of the quite considerable pressure on the diaphragm. Concentration is upon sitting tall and gaining a complete but erect spinal twist. Hold the posture for about thirty seconds initially, concentrating on the spinal column.

Let go of the left foot and lift it over the right thigh; stretch the left leg straight, then stretch the right leg straight and relax. Repeat this pose exactly for the other side, so that the effect on the left and right sides is balanced up.

Effects

The effects of this posture are felt almost immediately as it increases vitality and well-being. This asana twists the spine to both sides, benefitting the spinal column and the sympathetic nervous system. The muscles of the shoulder and abdomen are massaged, while constipation and dyspepsia are relieved. This posture is specially good for the liver, spleen and kidneys. In the *Hatha pradipika* it says that the Matsyendrasana rouses the Kundalini and stabilises the chandra. (At the biological level the chandra indicates the choroid plexus and the cerebal spinal fluid.)

Ardhamatsyendra

Ardha means 'half' and *matsyendra* we have already defined. This is a slightly easier form of the Matsyendrasana.

Method

Sit on the ground with your legs stretched out in front of you. Raise your right knee and bring your right foot up to the level of your left knee, keeping your right foot flat on the ground. Bring your left foot under your right leg and place it beneath your right buttock; keep your left knee flat on the ground and your body weight will be slightly shifted towards your left buttock. Bring your right foot over your left thigh and pull your foot back towards your body, keeping your right foot flat on the ground. Tuck your right knee under your left armpit and hold your left foot with your left hand. Bring your right arm around your back and tuck your right hand into your waist. Look to the extreme right, sitting tall and straight. Keep your chin slightly down to maintain the upright position of your spine and gently use your right knee as a lever to help you twist slightly further around. Concentrate on the spine and hold the position for about twenty seconds at first, breathing gently.

Relax carefully; first take the right arm to your side and place the right hand on the floor to maintain your balance, then bring your left hand over and remove your right foot, taking it back over your left knee to the front position, and finally take your left foot out and stretch both your legs out in front of you, relaxed. Repeat this posture reversing right and left so that the stimulations and stresses are balanced.

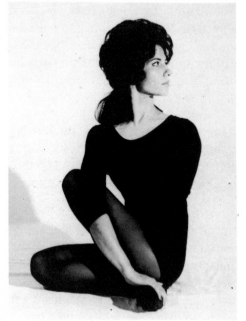

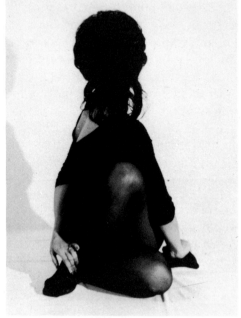

43 Ardha Matsyendrasana   44 Ardha Matsyendrasana

Effects

The effects are more or less the same as for the full Matsyendra posture, but the Ardhamatsyendrasana lacks the lower abdominal massage which the heel was able to give the lower intestines in the Matsyendrasana.

Trikonasana

Tri means 'three' and refers here to the idea of three inherent in time, ie past, present and future (this is called Kala in Sanskrit). *Kon* comes from a word meaning 'indifference', and *na* indicates a causal link. So *trikona* indicates an indifference to time, overcoming or making the passage of time superfluous and ineffective.

Method

Stand upright with your arms by your sides and your legs at an angle of sixty degrees apart, ie your feet should be the same distance apart as the length of your inner leg. Your feet should be facing straight forward and parallel to each other. Breathe in through your nose as you slowly raise your arms laterally to shoulder height; breathe out as you slowly bend forward and twist your trunk down to the left. Let your right hand touch the ground and bring it around until it is outside and behind your left foot with your fingers pointing to your back and your palm flat on the ground. Simultaneously raise the left arm vertically above you, turn your head to the left and look up at it (45). Hold your breath out in this position for about fifteen seconds, concentrating on the centre of your chest, and then slowly breathe in as you gradually stand up, keeping your feet in the same posi-

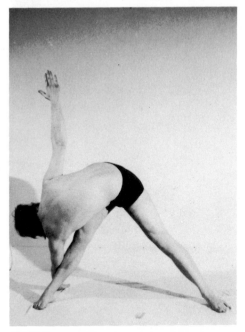

45 Trikonasana

tion and bringing your arms back to a lateral position at shoulder height. Repeat this exercise twisting to the right side. Finally breathe out and lower your arms to your sides and relax.

Effects

This makes the trunk of your body very supple and trims the waist. It has an effect upon the thymus through the movement of the rib cage and the intercostal muscles. It is the thymus which maintains youth and helps the body defences against infection; hence the name of this posture. This asana works on the Anhata Chakra.

Chandrasana

Chand means 'shine' and *ra* means 'having acquired, possessing or conferring'; thus chandra means 'that which has acquired a shining appearance. One of the signs of achievement in Hatha Yoga is a bright, shining appearance, and this is brought about by stimulation and cleansing of the nadis.

Method

Stand with your feet apart and your legs at an angle of sixty degrees. Your arms should be by your sides, your feet should be pointing forward and parallel. Breathe in as you raise your arms to shoulder height keeping them in the lateral line of your body precisely. Breathe out as you slowly bend to the right and place your right hand on your right ankle. As you do so, bring your left arm above your head, turning your left thumb under and back so that the left arm is locked straight, and bring the arm as far over your head towards the right as you can, feeling the pull on your left side. Look up towards your left hand (46). Hold your breath in this position for about fifteen seconds then slowly straighten up, breathing in at the same time. Repeat this exercise on the opposite side.

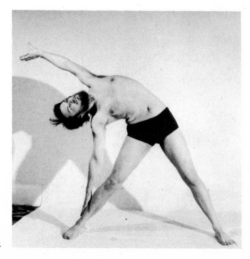

46 Chandrasana

Effects

This posture is very important in yoga practice and one of the few asanas which involve a sideways bend of the spine. Thus this posture is very beneficial for the spine, stimulating all the spinal nerves and, by reflex action, toning up the entire nervous system. It makes the spine supple and slims the waist while the sides of the body are stretched, thus removing psychosomatic tensions from those areas.

Padhastasana

Pad means 'foot' and *hast* means 'hand'. The Padhastasana is a posture which effectively helps the practiser to take the foot or basis of life in his own hands. The Sahasaram is enlivened and consciousness of real direction in life is produced. The personal energies associated with the Svadisthana Chakra are taken under control and used to manifest the direction of the higher levels.

Method

Stand upright with your feet together and arms by your sides. Breathe in as you raise your arms above your head and bend slightly backwards. Breathe out as you slowly bend forward from the lower sacral area and place your hands on either side of your feet. Make sure that your legs are straight. Hold your ankles with your hands and place your forehead on your shins (47). Hold your breath out in this position for about fifteen seconds. Slowly breathe in as, raising first your head and then your arms, you straighten up to the vertical position and relax.

Effects

This asana benefits the sacral area of the spine, strengthens the hamstrings and alleviates constipation. It works predominantly on the Svadisthana Chakra. Blood flows to the brain and the central nervous system is stimulated.

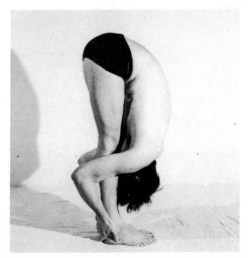

47 Padhastasana

Garudhasana

Garudha literally means 'eagle', but it is also the symbolic vehicle of Vishnu. In a creation myth it was Garudha who carried the meru mountain on its back to take it to the sea of milk in order to churn the sea to obtain amrit. Traditionally the eagle and the serpent are avowed enemies. The snake represents libido energy and the eagle is the symbol of elevated and sublimated sexual energy. The Garudhasana has received its name because it enables the practiser to put sexual energy to higher creative use.

Method

Stand straight with your feet together and arms by your sides. Transfer your weight to the left foot. Bring your right leg in front of your left thigh and bend your left knee slightly. Then bend your right knee and curl your right foot behind your left calf. Raise your right arm, with your elbow bent in a right angle and your right hand pointing upwards. Bend your left arm under your right arm and have your left hand crossed behind your right wrist; then bend your right wrist to cup over your left hand. Allow the tips of your fingers to touch your nose (48). Breathe gently in this posture and concentrate on balancing motionlessly while looking at a point on the ground about 10 ft in front of you. Hold this position for about thirty seconds and then relax gently, slowly straightening up. Repeat this exercise balancing on the right leg.

Effects

This posture, which works on the Muladhara Chakra, strengthens the knees and ankles and helps sterility and sexual debility. It puts pressure on the gonads and benefits the coccygeal nerves. It also improves balance and confidence.

48   Garudhasana

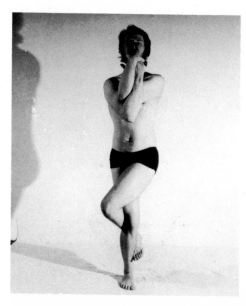

Natarajasana

This word comes from *nata* 'a dancer' and *raja* 'a lord'. This is one of the many names of Siva. The Natrajasana activates the Muladhara Chakra which is concerned with awareness of motion and rhythm. Hence this asana helps make us aware of the cosmic dance of the universe of vibration and energy. The creation of dance has been ascribed to Siva, who performed many dances in his icy home on Mount Kailash in the Himalayas and in the southern temple of Chidambaram. Of the one hundred or more dances he created, some are gently harmonious and peaceful, others fierce. The most famous of the terrible ones is the Tandava Nritya, or the cosmic dance of destruction. Siva, full of anger, dances to destroy his father-in-law, Daksha, who had been instrumental in causing the death of Siva's beloved wife, Sati. Siva, surrounded by his attendents, beats out a wild rhythm which threatens the world. Siva as Nataraja has inspired some of the finest Indian sculptures and bronzes. Hatha Yoga is also ascribed to Siva.

Method

Stand upright and transfer your weight to your right foot. Stretch your right arm out in front of your, keeping it parallel to the floor. Bend your left knee and, holding your left big toe between your index finger and left thumb, draw your left foot right up behind your back (49). Balance firmly for about fifteen seconds, breathing evenly and gently. Then release the grip on your leg and lower both arms to the sides. Repeat the posture for the right side.

Effects

This balancing posture develops grace and poise. It tones the leg muscles and is beneficial to all the vertebral joints.

49 Natarajasana

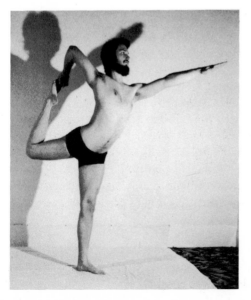

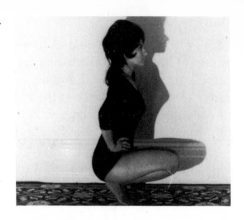

Angusthasana

Angusth is one of the sixteen adharas or vital points in the body. Of these angusth is the big toe.

Method

Stand with your feet together and transfer your weight to your toes. Slowly bend your knees, coming into a squat position with your knees and toes together. Place your hand on your hips and balance with your spine fairly upright (50).

Effects

This posture is an excellent complementary to the Vajrasana. The Vajrasana can become a little uncomfortable if it is held for too long, and the Angusthasana takes the strain out of the legs. In early practice, students often point their toes too much in postures such as the Sarvangasana and a mild form of cramp can often result. The Angustha posture removes the problem very quickly.

Ekapada Angusthasana

Eka means 'one' and *pada* is 'foot'. This posture is therefore, a variation of the angusthasana which envolves balancing on one foot only.

Method

Stand erect with your feet together and slowly raise your self until you are on the tips of your toes. Bend your knees and lower yourself until you are squatting on your heels (this is the Angusthasana). Make sure that your back is kept straight throughout. Carefully take your right foot and place it high across your left thigh. Put your hands on your hips and balance, breathing evenly and gently (51). (Concentration on a fixed point about 10ft away will help you balance.) Hold this position for about thirty seconds and then relax. Repeat this posture with the left side.

Effects

This exercise benefits the calf muscles and promotes psychological as well as physical balance through control of centres in the cerebellum.

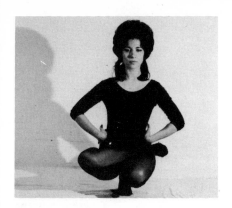

51   Eka Pada Angusthasana

Kakasana

Kak is the Sanskrit word for 'a crow'. As the crow takes any seeds that might have been carelessly sown by the farmer and consumes them, so the Kakasana disciplines the carelessly dispersed psychosexual energies (bindu) and frees the individual to discover the Self.

Method

Balance in the Angusthasana. Place your hands, palms downwards, flat on the ground in front of you with your fingers pointing forward. Bend your elbows slightly so that they touch the insides of your knees. Breathing in, gently lean forward and take the weight of your body on your hands. Let your upper arms press against your thighs (52). Balance in this position for about thirty seconds while holding your breath and then relax, breathing out.

Effects

This posture strengthens the wrists and benefits the thighs. It stimulates the sciatic nerves and tones up the pelvic nerves and related organs.

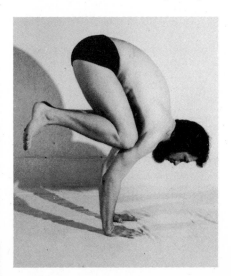

52   Kakasana

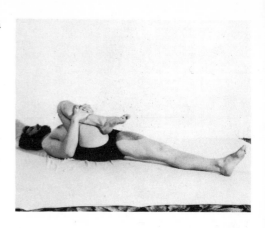

Vatnyasana

Vat is one of the humours of ancient Indian medicine. Vat, pitta and kapha are associated with the three outlets for products and toxins from the body. *Pitta* is usually translated as 'bile' or better, as 'metabolism' and *kapha* as 'phlegm', but a more worthy translation would go beyond this. *Vat* may be translated as 'wind', although a simple understanding of this would be misleading. The Vatnyasana is a posture which will effectively help you get rid of your wind.

Method

Lie flat on your back with your arms by your side. Breathe in and lift your right leg, bending it at the knee. Take hold of your knee with both hands and hold your breath in as you press the leg into your body for a few seconds (53). Relax and breathe out gently. Repeat this for the left side and then repeat the whole process once or twice more.

Effects

This cures flatulence and other wind disorders and benefits the abdomen.

Virabhadrasana

Bhadra has already been defined as 'auspicious, happy' and *vira* means 'hero' or 'brave'. The Bhadrasana gives the practiser confidence and removes psychosomatic personality blocks, which leaves you happier and more assured.

Method

Stand with your feet about 4-5ft apart. Turn to the right and point your right foot the way you are facing, keeping the left foot at right angles to it. Bend the right knee to form a right angle. Stretch the left leg back as far as possible keeping the left knee straight. Look straight ahead and stretch the spine back from the coccyx (54). Leave the arms loosely by the sides and maintain balance for about twenty to thirty seconds, breathing gently throughout. Place your hands on your knee to help you stand up carefully, and then relax. Repeat this posture on the other side.

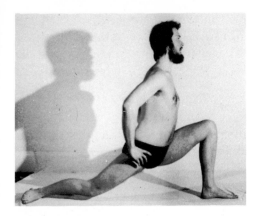

54 Vira Bhadrasana

Effects

This posture tones up the ankles and knees, removes stiffness from the lower back and reduces fat around the hips.

Anjaneyasana

This posture is also known as the Hanumanasana. Hanuman was the name of a powerful monkey chief who was the son of Anjana and the devoted friend and servant of Rama, the seventh incarnation of Vishnu. Once Laksman, Rama's brother, was injured by a karmic arrow in one of life's battles. The only cure was the juice of a herb which grew in the Himalayas. Anjaney (Ajana's son, Hanuman) leaped into a higher state of consciousness, symbolised by the mountain, and found a cure for Laksman in that state.

This posture is so named because it leads to a mental freeing from the physical/sexual world and the practiser is enabled to leave that world to 'leap' into a higher state of awareness.

Method

Kneel on the floor and put your palms down on the floor on either side of your body. Lift the knees and bring the right leg forward and take the left leg back. Try to stretch both legs straight with an exhalation, bearing your weight on your hands. Breathe in and repeat but bringing the other leg forward. This might

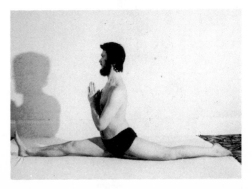

55 Anjaneyasana

take some time to do comfortably, but once you can rest the length of both legs on the floor (55) fold your hands in front of you and balance in this position for about thirty seconds, breathing gently. Then twist to one side and carefully bring your legs together into a sitting position. Repeat alternately bringing each leg in front.

Effects

This very graceful posture helps cure sciatica and tones and strengthens the leg muscles. It removes psychosomatic tensions from the area of the perineum.

Krounchasana

Krouncha is the Sanskrit word for 'a heron', but is also the name of a mountain, said to be the grandson of Himalaya, which was conquered by Kartikeya, the God of war, and Parsurama, the sixth incarnation of Vishnu. It brings a higher state of consciousness (Krouncha) which may be reached by removing psychosomatic tensions and freeing consciousness from the lower areas of the spine.

Method

Sit upright on the floor with your legs stretched out in front of you. Bend the right knee and place the right foot by the side of the right hip. The inner side of the right calf will touch the outer side of the right thigh. Breathe in, hold your breath and, taking hold of the left foot (making sure the left leg is straight), raise it so that the shin is touching your nose (56). Maintain this posture for ten seconds and then bring your left leg down, breathing out as you do so. Repeat this raising the other leg.

Effects

This eases the hamstrings in the legs and relieves tension in the lower sacral region.

56   Krounchasana

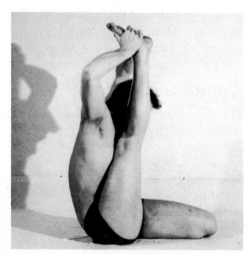

124

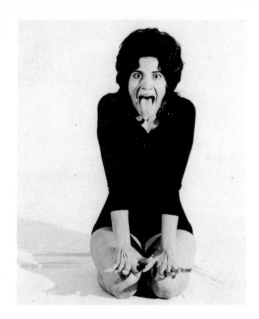

Simbhasana

This posture is called Simbhasana because it awakens our mind and we become like an alert lion who exhibits relaxed confidence.

Method

Sit in the Vajrasana. Put your hands on your knees and extend your fingers. Keeping your arms straight, lean forward slightly and put your tongue out and down as far as you can. Widen your eyes and imagine that you are a lion about to spring. Tense your neck, fingers and tongue and intensify the pose (57). Hold the posture for about five seconds, then relax.

Effects

This posture massages parts of the body which are normally neglected; the neck, root of the tongue, fingers and eyes benefit from it. Hearing is improved and the throat is cleansed. Consciousness is stimulated by reflex action through the effects this posture has on the cranial nerves.

Uttitha Kummerasana

Uttitha means 'raised' and *kummer* means 'waist' (as in cummerbund). It is simply a posture where the waist is raised.

Method

Kneel with your knees a few inches apart. Place your hands, palms down, on the ground about 2ft in front of your knees. Raise your back to its greatest extent whilst holding your breath and hang your head down between your arms (58). Then relax your back, breathing out as your raise your head (59). Repeat two or three times. This posture should be practised after the Dhanurasana.

125

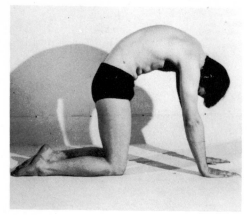
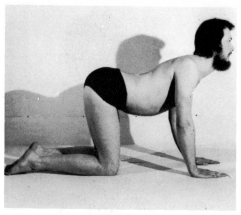

58 Uttitha Kummerasana stage 1   59 Uttitha Kummerasana stage 2

Effects

This pose relaxes the back and relieves back fatigue. It is an excellent exercise to perform during all stages of pregnancy.

Eye Exercises

Method

Sit in the Vajrasana, making sure that your spine is erect.

1   Look straight in front of you and then slowly and deliberately revolve your eyes from left to right in a circular motion; now blink slowly in an exaggerated way. Repeat the exercise from right to left and finish with a blink.

2   Look to the front and then move the eyes to the left as far as you can without turning your head; again look to the front, then move the eyes to the right and finally back to the front. Look up, then front again, look down and back to the front. Finish the exercise with a blink.

3   Looking straight ahead, raise your index finger to a point about 10in in front of your eyes and on level with them. Look at your finger and then at a point some distance behind it but at the same level. Look at your finger and then at the far point six or seven times in fairly rapid succession, focusing clearly each time. Finish the exercise by blinking.

Effects

These eye exercises will benefit the muscles which move your eyes and will also relieve eyestrain. In time, long- or short-sight problems will be corrected by working on the little muscles which accommodate your vision.

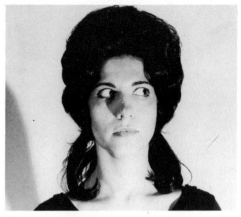

60   Second eye exercise

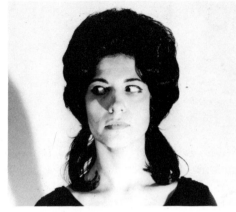

61   Second eye exercise

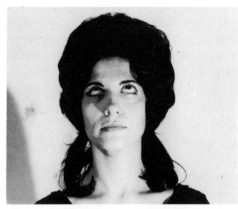

62   Second eye exercise

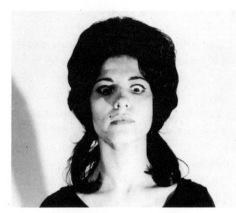

63   Second eye exercise

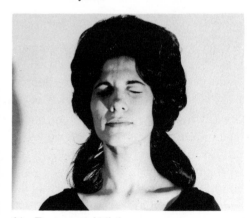

64   Exaggerated blink

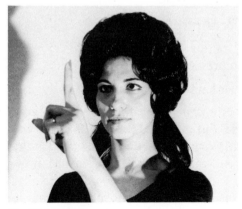

65   Third eye exercise

10 Mudras

Mudra is the body language of yoga. In everyday life we are continually communicating with body language, although not everyone is fully aware of it. Our hands and arms move and gesticulate when we speak, our facial muscles bring about all kinds of expressions—smiling, frowning—clearly reflecting our emotional and cognitive states. We stand tall and open when we are happy and full of energy. When we are depleted of energy and feeling unwanted or depressed, we droop our shoulders and bend forward and slouch. If you want to experience what another person is feeling, copy their posture and stance, make the same kind of facial expression, mimic them exactly and you will be able to penetrate their inner world completely and share their experiences and feelings.

Body and limb movements are great instructors, for they can teach us things that cannot always be communicated in words. For example, try to describe a spiral staircase and you are very likely to find yourself gesticulating within a few moments. Children everywhere learn from adults through imitating the way adults hold themselves, move and gesture.

There are countless mudras, all communicating something special. In yoga, a mudra is considered to be an expression of Kundalini energy moving through the body. By deliberately adopting certain mudras you may gain valuable experiences.

Brahma Mudra

Brahma is the name of the creator in the Trinity of Hindu philosophy. He is represented as having four heads.

Method

Sit in the Vajrasana. Place your fingers between your insteps behind your back, so that the shoulders are straight without being tense. Turn your head slowly to the right without moving your trunk; the chin should be brought almost in line with the right shoulder (66). Maintain this for five seconds and then turn your head so that you are looking straight in front of you. Repeat in the same way for the left side (67), pausing for about five seconds between movements and return to the original position. Bend your head backwards so that the muscles of the neck are stretched to a maximum without strain (68). Follow this by bringing the head forward and pressing the chin on the jugular notch (69). Again come back to the original position. Throughout the exercise concentrate on the area where the stretch is felt.

128

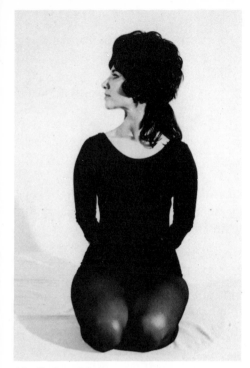

66 Brahma Mudra

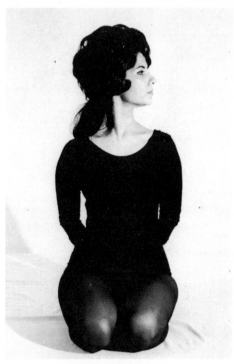

67 Brahma Mudra

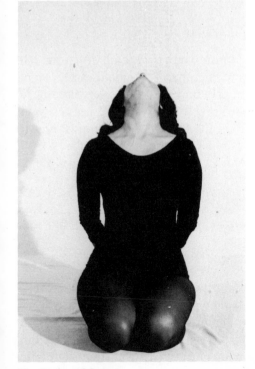

68 Brahma Mudra

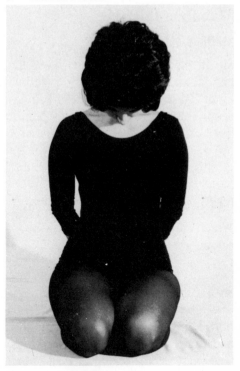

69 Brahma Mudra

Effects

Though the Brahma Mudra looks simple, it is an excellent exercise for removing psycho-physiological tensions. It stimulates the carotid nerve and arteries and gently works on the spinal nerves of the cervical area.

Special note: Beginners may keep their eyes closed during the posture to avoid eye strain.

Yoga Mudra

Method one

Sit in the Padmasana; place your clenched fists on your thighs on top of your feet. Breathe in and bend forward so that your forehead touches the floor (70). Maintain the position for as long as you can and then sit up, breathing out.

Method two

Sit in the Padmasana with your hands clasped behind your back. Breathe in and bend forward until your forehead touches the ground (71). Hold the posture for as long as you comfortably can and then sit up, slowly breathing out.

Effects

This exercise relieves constipation and improves digestion.

Mahabandha

Method

Sit in the Padmasana; cross your hands behind your back and with your left hand take hold of your left toes and with your right hand take hold of your right toes (72). If you breathe out as you do so you will find it a little easier. Breathe in deeply, then breathe out as you bend forward slowly from the hips and rest your head on the floor. Hold this mudra for about fifteen or twenty seconds. Slowly breathe in as you sit up, release you hands, undo your legs, and relax.

This mudra is completely self-contained and will itself teach you its meaning.

Maha Mudra

Maha means 'great' and the Maha Mudra is of great physical and spiritual value.

Method

Sit on the floor with your legs stretched straight out in front of you. Bend your left leg at the knee and set your heel against your perineum with the help of your right hand. Make sure your genitals do not get in the way. The sole of your left foot should be in close contact with your right thigh. Do not sit on your heel but have your heel pressing into the bone of your perineum. Bend over slightly to take hold of your right foot with both hands just below your toes, keeping your

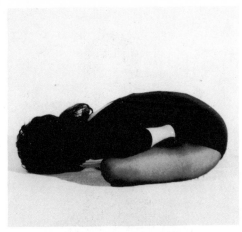

70　Yoga Mudra method one

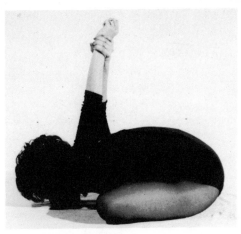

71　Yoga Mudra method two

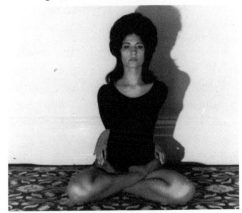

72　Mahabandha

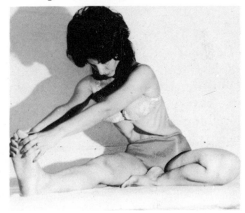

73　Maha Mudra

right foot vertical (73). Breathe in through both nostrils as you do in the Ujjayi technique and practise Kumbhakh. Perform the Uddiyani, Muladhara and Jalandhara bandhas whilst you are holding your breath. Relax the bandhas, breathe out gently, and sit up. Remove your left leg and relax. The mudra should be repeated with the left leg outstretched.

Effects

This mudra generates nervous activity which awakens the CNS and shows up in EEG recordings like the massive brainwaves of grand mal seizures.

Yoni Mudra

Method

Sit in the Padmasana and raise your hands to your face with your elbows at shoulder level. Put your thumbs in your ears and press slightly to cut off external sounds. Close your eyes and place your index fingers over your eyelids. Press gently towards the bottom of the eyeball. Breathe in and hold your breath as you

131

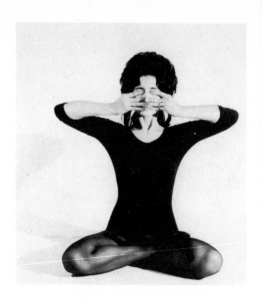

place your middle fingers on the side of your nose. Press your nostrils, gently closing them. Place your third fingers over the top of your upper lip and your fourth fingers underneath your lower lip. Gently press your third and fourth fingers together thus closing your lips. Hold the mudra for as long as you comfortably can and then remove your fingers and breathe gently, relaxing. Repeat the whole exercise.

Whilst in this mudra you will soon hear a kind of whistling or ringing sound filling your head. Listen to the subtler tones and gradually the ringing will become greater and greater. This sound is called the nada, and is rather like a homing beacon. It informs you that you are beginning to awaken, and if you concentrate completely on it you will find that you go beyond the senses to a high state of meditation. This technique will lead you very naturally into the Nada-bandha.

Effects

This mudra cuts out sensory information and stimulates the facial and other cranial nerves.

Aswini Mudra

Aswini means 'of a mare' and the Aswini Mudra may well be named from its resemblance to the contractions and dilations of the anal aperture of a mare which are usually observable when it runs.

Method

Contract your anal sphincter and, in conjunction with the muscles of the pelvis, contract your anal region upwards and inwards, then consciously relax it. In females this process is even more complex and includes contractions of the vagina. Initially it may be easier to contract and relax the anal region in tune with a rhythmic breathing; with some practice, however, the contractions may be performed independently of your breathing rhythm. After considerable practice you will be able to perform this mudra in any position. In the early stages it is best done lying on your back, drawing your folded legs up towards your body. The Aswini Mudra may be performed during certain asanas; for example, it may be usefully performed in Viparita Karna and during the Vatnyasana.

Effects

Apart from its psychological advantages, this mudra also tones up the pelvic muscles and counteracts constipation, prolapse and piles.

Khechari Mudra

This is a very famous technique indeed, but it is often totally misunderstood. It is said that the Khechari Mudra involves cutting, manipulating and milking the tongue so that it gradually lengthens until it can touch the middle of the eyebrow. According to this interpretation the operation should be carried out with a sharp, clean knife, the shape of a milk hedge leaf. Each day you should cut the frenum to a hair's breadth and rub it with rock salt. After seven days you should cut it again and this process should be repeated until the frenum is severed. Then the tongue is turned back into the place of the junction of the three paths. The three paths are the Ida, Pingala and Sushumna, or in modern neural terms the parasympathetic, sympathetic and central nervous systems. They meet at the level of the hypothalamus which composes the floor of the third ventricle. This is called Khechari Mudra. In the *Hathapradipika* it says that the yogi who remains with his tongue turned upwards for even half a kshana (the smallest fraction of time, a moment), is freed from disease, death and old age, and cannot be poisoned. He who practises the Khechari Mudra escapes from premature death, fatigue, sleep, hunger, thirst or stupor. He who masters the Khechari Mudra is not bound by karma or by time.

We have met a number of practitioners of the literal technique of Khechari Mudra and have not been impressed by their yogic attainments. We do not believe that the Khechari Mudra is intended to be taken literally, in the physical sense, and we return to the original Sanskrit text to solve the problem. *Khechari* literally means 'moving in space' and indicates a higher state of consciousness. The word that is normally translated as 'tongue' is *rasana*, but this is not the normal word used for the physical, muscular tongue. It means something more like 'the experiencer'. Thus our translation of the original runs as follows:

When the taster of experience, Rasana (symbolised by the tongue), is severed from the root of experience, the senses, by the sharp instrument of the intellect, the experience of the pure existence of the void is attained.

Consciousness (Brahman) is most clearly experienced by concentrating on the third ventricle of the brain, which was called the cave of Brahman by the ancient rishis. The stream of juice which is said to be continually produced by an organ called the chandra is said to have all tastes, and indeed the yogi should have tasted life fully. Experience is the great teacher, and through learning all that life has to offer the yogi can no longer be disturbed, but becomes a source of understanding and wisdom for all. In the physical body the Chandra is the choroid plexus which produces cerebrospinal fluid. By directing your experience to the third ventricle and concentrating on that area in the centre of your head, you will experience a very high state of meditation beyond the senses. Khechari Mudra, then, is the directing of your attention up into the centre of your head.

In the third ventricle there is no nervous material, and by concentrating on that point you may have the experience of nothing. You will literally be moving, being in the nothing. The experience of nothing is Yoga—the state where neither the experiencer nor the experience exists separately. This achievement undoubtedly exists in the attainments listed in the *Hathapradipika* and elsewhere.

There are also a number of secondary mudras, two of which are described here:

Bhoomi Sparsh Mudra

Bhoomi means 'earth' and *sparsh* means 'to touch'.

Method

Sit in the Padmasana. Place the tips of your index fingers against the tips of your thumbs. Lightly rest your palms on your knees to that the tips of your remaining fingers touch the ground.

This is a good posture for meditation or composure as it puts you in contact with the earth's pranic fields. Buddha is traditionally depicted in this pose.

Jnana Mudra

Jnana means 'knowledge'.

Method

Sit in the Padmasana, making sure that your spine is erect. Curl your index finger, which represents the ego, into the thumb, which represents the will (both hands). Place your hands on your knees so that the palms face upwards. This posture is traditionally used for meditation.

11 Bandhas

All human beings tend to have anal and sexual difficulties, problems with speech and thought, and communication blocks at individual, social, national, international and cosmic levels. One may overcome these problems by practising the five bandhas—Mula, Uddiyana, Jalandhara, Nada and Brahma. These bandhas are also incorporated into certain asanas and are practised during Kumbakh in Pranayama. Some other useful bandhas are also described in this chapter.

Mulabandha

Mula means 'root' or 'source' and Mulabandha is an exercise which works mainly on the lowest portion of our body—the pelvis—to affect the central and sympathetic nervous systems through the nerves which terminate there. Through practice of Mulabandha the yogi reaches towards the source (mula) of creation, rather than dwelling in the realm of the psycho-sexual and material which is the root of all frustration and dissatisfaction.

Method

Sit on a comfortable posture, such as Padmasana, Siddhasana or Sukhasana. Contract the anal and lower pelvic muscles. There are two anal muscles—known as sphincters—one internal and the other external, both situated at the end of the rectum. Both of these should be contracted and so should the whole of the pelvic region. Withdraw psychic energy from the lower part of your abdomen and draw apana force upwards.

Effects

A great deal of psychic energy and awareness is often invested in the sexual organs, and a method for controlling sexual stimulation is necessary if this energy is to be released for higher work. Mulabandha opens the way for the development of ojas power—hormonal power which can be used for physical, mental and spiritual development.

If sexual energy is misused or not properly controlled, it will be so depleted that eventually you may become impotent and be unable to obtain sexual satisfaction. By controlling apana force, which normally tends to move in a downward direction, you may maintain a high sexuality and orgastic potential.

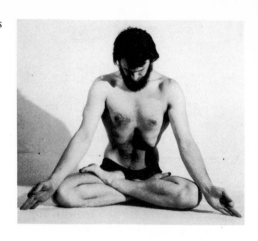

Uddiyanabandha

Uddiyana means 'to fly up'. When this bandha is practised, energy is moved from the abdominal regions and 'flies up' through the Sushumna—the central nervous system.

Method

Uddiyana should be performed only when the stomach is empty. Either stand squarely and comfortably, leaning forward slightly and resting your hands on your knees, or sit in a comfortable posture. Exhale completely, close your glottis, and hold your breath throughout. Fix your shoulders and clavicle firmly by pressing your hands against your knees. Lift up your rib cage by contracting the intercostal muscles. This increases the capacity of the thorax and thus air pressure becomes negative; the diaphragm, which is already relaxed after expiration, rises still higher in the thoracic cavity. At the same time as the ribs are raised, the front abdominal muscles are completely relaxed, and the abdomen takes on a concave appearance (75). Uddiyana should be held for about one minute and then relaxed. Initially it can be repeated four or five times.

Effects

The abdominal muscles are drawn upwards and backwards, producing a squeezing effect on the abdominal organs. Their hormones, which are concerned with metabolic processes, are secreted into the bloodstream. It has an excellent effect on the digestion and can help relieve disorders of the alimentary tract. Uddiyana practice will soon banish constipation and will effect a positive improvement in most chronic abdominal diseases.

Uddiyana is the mother of Nauli, which is dealt with in the section on kriyas.

Jalandharabandha

The word *jala* refers to the brain and the nerves passing through the neck, and dhara refers to the afferent flow of information to the brain.

136

Method

Place the chin on the chest, either in the jugular notch or a little below it, contract the throat and close the vocal cords, which are situated in the larynx. Tighten the muscles of the neck and press the chin on to the chest as firmly as possible.

Effects

Jalandhara achieves its effects by exerting pressure on the carotid sinus. The carotid sinus is a dilation at the bifurcation of the common carotid artery which has two branches, the internal and external carotid artery. These arteries are situated on both sides of the neck and are mainly responsible for bringing blood supply to the brain. The carotid sinus is usually restricted to the first part of the internal carotid. The walls of the sinus are thin and easily yield to internal or external pressure.

The sinus nerve is a branch of a cranial nerve coming from the brain (see Chapter 5). Rising just below the skull, it descends on the internal carotid artery and is distributed to the wall of the carotid sinus. If pressure is applied externally to the carotid sinus, the sinus nerve is stimulated and nerve impulses travel to the brain producing a general trance-like state which has the effect of slowing down the heart. This was well-known to the ancient rishis who called the sinus nerve *vijrianadi*—the nerve of consciousness.

In the performance of Jalandhara, the closure of the glottis, the tightening of the neck muscles and the sharp bend of the neck all contribute to exert considerable pressure on the carotid sinus so that the carotid nerve is stimulated. In this contraction the thyroid gland is activated and hormones which direct metabolism, energy, growth and nutrition are secreted into the bloodstream.

Through constant practice this bandha can be perfected until one is able to withdraw from sensory awareness in a controlled manner.

During Pranayama, when the breath is retained for a long time after deep inhalation it is possible for the pent up air in the lungs to rush out through the Eustachian canals to the internal ear and thus lead to various disorders. By the practice of Jalandhara during Kumbakh this undesirable possibility is guarded against.

Nadabandha

Nadabandha is practised with Yoni Mudra as indicated in Chapter 10. Total concentration on the experience of nada (sound current) at the centre of the head behind the eyes is called the Nadabandha. With this technique the breath can be virtually stopped and the personality absorbed in the cosmic ocean of vibration and music.

Brahmabandha

When, through absolute concentration on the nada current, the personality is completely absorbed and no separation at all is experienced, the transcendental

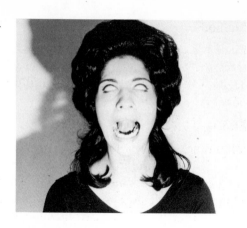

Self—Brahman—is alone. Respiration and other metabolic processes cease. The separated ego disappears, just as a cup of water disappears when it is thrown into the ocean.

Jihvabandha

Jihva means 'the tongue' or 'individual' and Jihvabandha is the tongue lock.

Method

The upper surface of the tongue is tightly pressed against the hard and soft palates (76).

Effects

Through a reflex action via the cranial nerves that innervate the tongue, the mind is awakened the sound of the nada current is increased and you will become more aware of your individuality.

Viparitakarni

Viparita means 'inverted' and *karni* means 'action'; thus the Viparitakarni is simply the 'inverted action'.

Method

Lie flat on your back on the ground with your legs straight and together. Slowly raise your legs from the hips, keeping your knees straight. Support your hips with your hands and rest your weight on your elbows. Raise your trunk to an angle of about forty five degrees with the ground and maintain your legs at right angles to your body (77). Notice that the chin is away from the chest in this position. Remove your arms and place them flat on the ground. Perform the Jihvabandha in this position whilst visually concentrating on your toes. Maintain this exercise for about twenty seconds at first; later, according to the advice of your teacher, you may increase the time considerably, but not beyond twenty minutes even when advanced. If this exercise is practised with a succession of others as part of a programme, about six minutes is optimal.

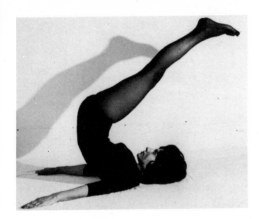

77 Viparita Karni

Effects

The upper part of the body and the brain are flushed with blood and the brain, medulla oblongata and spinal nerves etc are toned up.

Bandhas and Dharana techniques may be used in Vipontakami to modify hormone production and cerebrospinal fluid composition. As an inverted exercise electromagnetic influences of the environment on the body are altered and generally have a rejuvenating effect.

12 Pranayama

Traditionally there are said to be 72,000 Pranayama exercises. Many of the Pranayama techniques are also breathing techniques but it should not be thought that Pranayama is simply concerned with physical breathing; it is a necessary life process. As we saw earlier, *pranayama* means 'expansion of energy'. In the *Hathapradipika* it says that even Brahma and the other gods devoted themselves to the practise of Pranayama to free themselves from the fear of death[1]. Pranayama expands us beyond our communication clocks, freeing us from our limited body image. It is said that the impurities of the nadis are removed by Pranayama alone and by no other means.

The ultimate in Pranayama is Kevali Kumbhak. This Kumbhak is practised when holding of the breath is preceded by neither Purakh nor Rechakh. In perfect concentration, the breath does stop, as has been demonstrated by yogis under exacting conditions.

The following Pranayama methods have been selected as representative of their kind. They are normally practised in the order listed below:

Simple pranayama
Suryabhedana
Ujjayi
Sitkari
Sitali
Bhastrika
Bhramari
Murccha

Simple Pranayama

Simple Pranayama is the basis of all Pranayama techniques.

Method

Sit in a comfortable posture. Close your right nostril with your right thumb and slowly inhale through the left nostril for the count of three. Fill your entire chest with air. Retain your breath for the count of twelve, concentrating on the point above and between your eyebrows, and close your left nostril with the ring and fourth finger of your right hand. Remove your thumb and exhale through your right nostril slowly and steadily for the count of six. Breathe in through your right nostril for the count of three. Close the right nostril with your thumb and

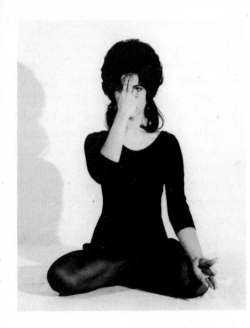

retain the breath for the count of twelve, keeping both nostrils closed with thumb and ring finger. Remove your ring finger and little finger from your left nostril and slowly breath out for the count of six. Normally, bandhas are performed during the kumbhak stage.

This is one round of pranayama. Rather like a round of sandwiches which contains two slices of bread, one round of alternate nostril breathing includes two complete breaths. Three rounds should be performed in the initial stages and this may be increased by one round a week according to the directions of your teacher. As part of a daily yoga session, sixteen rounds of pranayama taking about twenty-five minutes to perform would constitute a typical medium level programme.

Effects

Alternate nostril breathing tones up the autonomic nervous system and produces a feeling of expansion and lightness. It is a great healing technique and considerably helps the development of concentration. The nerves lining the sinuses and nasopharyngeal cavities are selectively stimulated in this exercise. Nervous impulses relayed to the central nervous system may programme the CNS like a computer to achieve specific desired effects.

Suryabhedana

Surya means 'sun' and the word is used here to represent the right nostril and the sympathetic nervous system. *Bhedana* means 'opening out, blooming, piercing or breaking through', and thus Suryabhedana is the pranayama which is used for awakening the Kundalini and in which inhalation is made through the right nostril.

Method

Sit in a firm, comfortable position which can be maintained for a long time without discomfort. Slowly inhale air through the right nostril, closing the left nostril with the ring and fourth finger of the right hand. Retain the breath, closing your right nostril with your right thumb, until you feel pressure all over the body, extending even to the hair and ends of your nails. Having held the breath to capacity, slowly exhale through the left nostril. As with Simple Pranayama, the ratio of breathing-in time to holding-time to breathing-out time is 1:4:2. The beginner should start on a ratio of approximately 3 seconds: 12 seconds: 6 seconds. Although the student may feel capable of a longer time ratio the temptation to speed up progress should be avoided. The good yoga teacher wants the student to progress at the optimum speed but knows that short-cutting without experiential knowledge can be dangerous and is therefore to be avoided.

Purakha, Kumbhak and Rechakh form one round of Suryabhedana. Five rounds should be performed initially under the strict guidance of a teacher. This may normally be extended by one round each week until the timing of the breathing ratio is increased, when the number of rounds will be brought down.

Later, after reasonable practice. Suryabhedana should be performed with bandhas held during Kumbhak.

Effects

Suryabhedana increases digestive power (jathar agni), stimulates the sympathetic nervous system and cleans the sinuses. This technique has a considerable heating effect on the body, and heavy perspiration is likely.

Note: People who have low blood pressure will find this exercise of particular benefit, but anyone with high blood pressure should avoid the technique until they have brought their blood pressure down by other practices.

Ujjayi

U implies something superior, that which is above, while *jayi* indicates victory or overcoming. Ujjayi, then, is a superior Pranayama technique which enables the practitioner to overcome all diseases.

Method

Sit in a firm, comfortable posture. Inhale through both nostrils, producing a humming sound which can be felt from the throat to the heart. Retain the breath for four times the length of the inhalation. Perform Mulabandha Uddiyanabandha, and Jalandharabandha during Kumbhak. Relax the bandhas and breath out gently through the mouth, making the sound 'ha'. The air should be felt on the palate as it is expelled. The time taken to breathe out should be twice the inhalation time. This is one round of Ujjayi and about five rounds should be practised initially. Ujjayi may be practised whilst walking and at any time during the day.

142

Effects

Ujjayi has a general cleansing and toning-up effect on the whole body. Whilst the rate of breathing is markedly reduced by this technique, oxygen consumption usually increases by about 25 per cent over normal levels. Initially a sense of tingling may be experienced throughout the body, and after a little practice a state of cholinergia is produced, as the parasympathetic nervous system becomes dominant. Among cholinergic characteristics is a lowered blood pressure, and thus Ujjayi is most beneficial for people suffering from high blood pressure.

Sitkari

Sitkari means 'having or possessing' *sit*. *Sit* is a close approximation to the sound made during the Purakh stage of this pranayama. *Sit* also means 'cold'. Sitkari is thus the pranayama which causes coldness and makes the sound 'sit'.

Method

Sit in the normal way for Pranayama practice. Open your mouth a little by slightly dropping the lower jaw and raising the upper lip. Protrude your tongue slightly beyond your lower incisors and draw its tip inside to press against the incisor teeth. The sides of your tongue should cover your lower molars and premolars. Raise the lower jaw pressing your tongue lightly between your upper and lower molars and premolars. The padding of your tongue will leave a small opening between your front teeth through which air may be sucked producing the sound 'si'. After inhalation the mouth should be closed, and this tends to make the sound 't'. Retain the breath for four times the inhalation time, then breathe out evenly through the nose.

Repeat Purakh, Kumbhak and Rechakh for five rounds initially, in the same time ratio as in the other Pranayama techniques. Under qualified instruction you will be able to progress quite quickly in this exercise, as with the other pranayamas. Later, when you are ready, bandhas may be introduced during Kumbhak.

Effects

This technique has a cooling effect and is soothing to the eyes and ears. It will be found beneficial to those suffering from biliousness or mild fever. Sitkari stimulates the liver and spleen, improves digestion and relieves the psychological experience of thirst.

Sitali

The name Sitali is derived from the cooling effect which this pranayama has on the body.

Method

Sit in the usual way for Pranayama practice. Protrude your tongue about $\frac{3}{4}$in

143

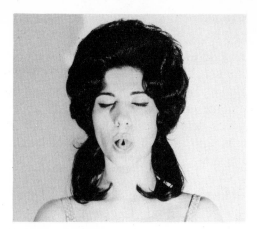

beyond your lips. Fold your tongue double along its length so it forms a channel (79); as the channel tends to narrow towards the tip of the tongue, it looks rather like the beak of a bird. Inhale air through the tube made by the tongue for the usual time. Practise retention, with your mouth closed, for four times the duration of inhalation. Breathe out evenly through your nostrils. This is one round of Sitali.

Start Sitali practice under the instruction of a teacher, beginning with five rounds and progressing as advised. Later, bandhas should be performed during Kumbhak.

Effects

Normally breath is inhaled through the nose and is moistened and warmed before entering the lungs. In Sitali the air is sucked in through the mouth and thus it produces a cooling effect. This practice should therefore not be carried out in very cold or very hot air, but in mild atmospheric conditions.

This exercise has a soothing effect on the eyes and ears. If suffering from biliousness or mild fever it can help relieve symptoms. Sitali has a positive aiding effect on the metabolic systems, activitating the liver and improving digestion.

Note: People with high blood pressure should practise initially without performing Kumbhak.

Bhastrika

Bhastrika means 'a bellows', a device used to force air in and out.

Method one

Sit firmly in the normal way. Breathe in and out evenly, rapidly and forcefully. This technique will be quite audible. The breath is moderately shallow and you should concentrate on your frontal sinuses. Rapid, even forceful, breathing through both nostrils should be practised for about ten to twelve cycles. Then take a deep, slow breath and retain it, practising Mulabandha for three seconds. Then breathe out gently and completely. Alternatively one round of Ujjayi may be performed. Repeat this practice about three times during early stages.

Method two

Practise rapid, forceful breathing through the right nostril only for about twelve cycles, closing the left nostril with the ring and fourth finger of the right hand. Repeat exactly the same process through the left nostril only, closing the right nostril with the right thumb. Inhale a complete breath through both nostrils, hold the breath, performing Mulabandha for two or three seconds, and then breathe out gently and fully or perform one round of Ujjayi. Repeat this cycle about three times more.

Effects

Bhastrika activates and invigorates the liver, spleen, pancreas and abdominal muscles. Digestion is improved and the sinuses are drained. The CNS is stimulated by a reflex action.

Bhramari

Bhramari is the Sanskrit word for 'a bee'. This pranayama is called Bhramari because when it is performed a sound rather like that of a bee is produced.

Method

Breathe in through the nose in such a way as to vibrate the soft palate and uvula. This is rather like the process of snoring, although in this case the sound is melodious and even, as against the rougher, disrupted sound made in snoring. As you breathe in you should feel the soft palate being drawn up towards the wall of the pharynx and vibrating to make a high-pitched humming noise. Inhale in this way for the normal time. Hold your breath for four times as long as your inhaling time performing the three bandhas and then breathe out through the nose. You should produce the same humming noise as during the inhalation, although the pitch will be slightly lower as the breath is exhaled more slowly, taking twice as long to exhale the breath as inhale.

Practice Purakh, Kumbhak and Rechakh about five times in this way when first starting.

Effects

This technique will bring great peace of mind and pleasurable sensations may well be felt in various parts of the body. It helps lull insomniacs to sleep.

Murccha

This pranayama is called *Murccha,* meaning 'unconsciousness', because it leads to a loss of awareness and a stupor which is both instructive and pleasant. Such a loss of awareness could be brought about by drugs, but here it is done independently, thus avoiding physical, psychological and social side effects. This technique should be practised under the supervision of a good teacher and, as with drugs, it should not be experimented with casually.

Method

Sit in a firm, comfortable posture where you will not overbalance. Inhale deeply through both nostrils. Perform Kumbhak with Jalandhara Bandha. The bandha should be held very strongly during an extended retention of breath and even maintained during Rechakh phase. Continued performances of a large number of rounds will lead to a loss of perceptual awareness and a resulting exclusion of sensory disturbance. Great concentration and directed effort is required to perform Murccha properly. Consciousness is maintained throughout, it is only the objects of consciousness which are excluded in this technique. Improper and unattentive attempts to practise Murccha will lead to fainting which is not the objective and is more or less useless for Pranayama purposes.

Various forms of Dharana may be performed during this practice.

Through pranayama practice you will become aware of bioenergetic pathways (nadis) which are not the same as the physical pathways of the body, but are part of the bioenergetic body known as the pranamaya kosha. You will be able to direct your pranas through those channels at will to achieve various yogic effects eg pranic healing, psychokinesis.

13 Kriyas

The kriyas (*kriya* means 'action') are also called the Shatkarmas. *Shat* means 'six' and *karma* also means 'action'. The Shatkarmas are six practices which can help to cure mental and physical disease. These techniques are not required by someone in perfect health but they are included as part of yoga practice because sometimes students make mistakes in their practice and become ill. This is very unlikely if you have a good teacher, but if you are egotistical and think that you can practise yoga without a teacher then you suffer ill-effects. Yoga techniques cannot be learned from a book but only from a teacher. Do not attempt to practise any of these techniques without a good teacher.

In the *Hathapradipika*[1] it says that anyone who has an excess of fat or phlegm should practise the six purificatory processes before commencing any of the other yoga practices. The six purificatory processes are Dhauti, Basti, Neti, Nauli, Tratakam and Kapalabhati. These six actions should be carefully kept secret as they produce various remarkable results and are held in great esteem.

Dhauti

Method

Dhauti is the basic yoga technique for cleaning the stomach internally by means of swallowing a cloth. The cloth should be made of fine muslin and be about 3in in breadth and about 23ft long. It must be soft or the alimentary tract will be in danger of being badly scratched. The cloth should be cleaned, washed and sterilised by boiling it for about ten minutes before use. You will find it best to roll the cloth up before starting the practice of Dhauti. To help the act of swallowing, the cloth should be first soaked in water and then lightly squeezed until it stops dripping. If it is too dry the cotton cloth will soon absorb saliva when it is introduced into the mouth, making swallowing very difficult; if it is too wet, the saliva will be diluted and again the act of swallowing will be very difficult.

The loose end of the cloth is held between the forefinger and the middle finger and then inserted into the throat as deep as the fingers can go. You then swallow it just as you would swallow ordinary food. When you are sure that the throat has grasped the cloth you can continue to insert it bit by bit and can even begin to chew the cloth as you would ordinary mouthfuls of food, although this must be done gently in order to avoid breaking it. You are really mimicking ordinary eating and dealing with the cloth just as you would deal with eating bread and butter.

Do not try to eat too much on the first day. The tender mucous membranes

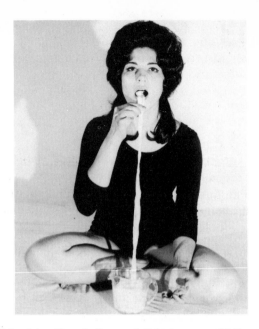

which line the throat are constantly rubbed by the cloth, and this leaves a little soreness because of the friction. On the first day you should only eat about 12-16in. After about a fortnight's practice the membrane becomes accustomed to this kind of rubbing and the soreness disappears. An extra 12 or 16in may be eaten every day so that after about fifteen days the entire length of cloth can be swallowed.

Most people of average health will find that the practice of Dhauti causes them few problems, but people with throat conditions or hypersensitive throat linings will find that even the very touch of the cloth is liable to provoke violent coughing. The eyes can become reddened and filled with tears, the nose is liable to run and the practitioner is likely to despair of ever achieving proper Dhauti. With a good teacher, however, all these problems will be overcome after two or three attempts. Many people find that the process of swallowing is made easier by soaking the cloth in milk. This tends to increase the secretion of saliva which in turn makes the cloth rather more slimy so that it slides down the throat more easily. In some cases even a little sugar may be added to the milk, but after some practice the amount of sugar and milk may be progressively reduced until Dhauti can be performed without difficulty. Occasionally some difficulty is experienced in practising Dhauti and there may be a tendency to retch. When this happens you should simply shut your mouth and keep perfectly passive. After two or three spasms your system will settle down and you will be ready to carry on swallowing.

Make sure you keep at least 8in of the cloth outside your mouth so that there is no danger of the other end being drawn into the stomach; moreover you need this amount to help pull the cloth out. Uddiyana and Nauli may be practised whilst the cloth is in your stomach. The cotton cloth tends to absorb fluids which

148

have collected in the stomach and the walls of the stomach sit tight on the cloth, churning it by their involuntary actions. Thus the stomach is gently rubbed against the cloth and a sort of massage is carried out. The time spent in swallowing is not as important as the time the cloth is allowed to remain in the stomach. It should not be left there more than about twenty minutes, otherwise the cloth is in danger of being passed on out of the stomach through the pyloric sphincter. If this is allowed to happen injury to the pyloric sphincter and perhaps to the intestines is possible.

Withdrawal of the cloth does not require much technique as it becomes so slippery that it can easily be pulled out. A gentle, steady pull with the mouth gaping wide open is the best technique. If the cloth is held back, as can sometimes happen, you should retract a few inches of it and, with the mouth shut, keep perfectly passive for a few seconds. Your whole system will adjust and you will then be able to continue the withdrawal. The cloth should be collected in a basin.

A teaspoon of clarified butter may be taken after the practice.

If you find you get a very sore throat through practising this you should suspend your practice of Dhauti for a few days and take it up later when your throat has returned to normal.

Under proper instruction there is little that can go wrong in Dhauti. One of the few problems that can arise is that the cloth may snap. If this does occur, an emetic should be taken, such as common salt water, and the cloth will soon be regurgitated. Obviously Dhauti should be practised on an empty stomach, and the best time is in the morning. During practice of Dhauti the diet should be carefully controlled; sour, pungent and sharp foods particularly should be avoided and intake of milky, creamy foods and clarified butter should be increased.

Effects

Dhauti cures all gastro-intestinal diseases.

Basti

Basti means 'washing' and there are a number of variations of Basti. Uttarabasti is the practice of washing the sex organs and Adhobasti is the practice of washing the rectum and the anal canal. These are the two main practices. Netrabasti is the cleansing of the eyes with water and Karnabasti is the cleansing of the ears, but this should only be resorted to if there is a serious disorder of the ear.

Method: Uttarabasti

Briefly, Uttarabasti is performed by introducing pure water or milk into the urethra using a suitable syringe. Females may irrigate the entire vaginal tract with this technique using the Aswini Mudra (Chapter 10).

Effects

Uttarabasti has a beneficial effect on all genital disorders as well as ensuring cleanliness and thus preventing disease.

Method: Adhobasti

To perform Adhobasti you will need a piece of hose about 5in long with a central hole of less than ½in in diameter. Smear the end of the hose with a little oil or suitable ointment and introduce it into the anal canal, leaving about 1in protruding. Have your feet slightly apart and sit in the Angustha pose. You should do this in a bath of water which has been filled to knee height. Contract your abdomen rhythmically and draw water up into your anal passage. The contents of the rectum may then be expelled in the normal way. This process should be repeated three or four times. It is probably easier and more convenient for most students in the West to practise using an enema instead.

Effects

Adhobasti helps relieve all intestinal disorders, the senses are enlightened and digestion is improved.

Nauli

In some ways Nauli is considered to be an evolution of Uddiyanabandha.

Method

In the early stages Nauli is best practised standing up. Place your hands on your hips and bend your chest forward. Take a deep breath through your nose and then quickly breath out completely through your mouth. Close your mouth and do not breathe in. Contract your abdomen and stomach up and back underneath your rib cage so that you produce a hollow. Then contract the middle recti muscles which will stand out like a ridge down the centre of your abdomen. This is called Madhyanauli. Relax the muscles and then repeat this four or five times before completely relaxing and breathing in through the nose.

The next stage in the practice of Nauli is to contract and isolate the right and left recti alternately. The right rectus muscle contracted on its own is called Dakshinanauli and the left rectus contracted is called Wamanauli. With a little practice the two may be alternated and a churning effect is produced. Nauli may be practised with a clockwise or an anti-clockwise motion, and initially you should perform five or six rotations in one direction, relax, and then perform five or six rotations in the opposite direction.

Effects

Nauli helps relieve abdominal and chest disorders and stimulates the metabolism, giving perfect health.

Note: This exercise should not be attempted by people with acute abdominal conditions and must be avoided during all stages of pregnancy.

150

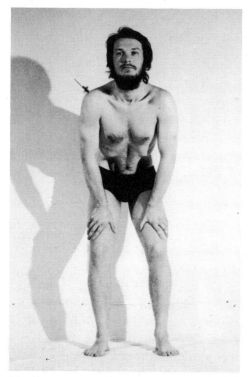

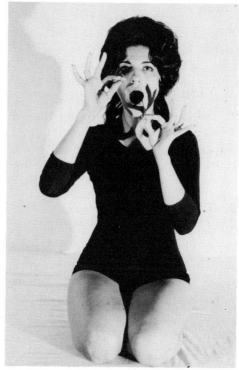

81 Nauli   82 Neti

Neti

Method

Take a cord of soft cotton thread about 16in long and dip one end of the cord into soft, hot, beeswax and cool it so as to make it slightly still but pliable. Widen your nostrils and introduce the waxed end of the cord into one nostril, closing the other nostril with your thumb. Breathe in rapidly and breathe out gently through the mouth, continuing until the cord appears in the back of the throat. Place your finger inside your mouth and bring the cord out through. Pull the cord through until the soft, unwaxed part of the cord lies in the nasal passage. Gently pull the cord to and fro five or six times (82) then remove the cord from your nasal passage through the mouth. With a clean cord, or after having washed the same cord, repeat this practice through the other nostril. In the West this process may be performed using a suitable rubber catheter.

A second method of performing Neti is called Jalaneti. Hold some tepid, slightly salty water either in the palms of your hands or in a suitable vessel and breathe the water up through one nostril, closing the other with your thumb. Tilt your head back and allow the water to come into your mouth. Do not swallow it but spit it out. Repeat the same process through the other nostril. This exercise can be combined with tilting the head to the left and right in order to allow the saline solution to run through the sinus and thus clean them also.

Effects

Neti cleans the entire head and, by reflex action, stimulates the whole nervous system. It destroys sinus and neck diseases and relieves a number of different kinds of headache,

Kapalbhati

Kapalbhati is often confused with Bhastrika—the bellows breath—which is a Pranayama technique. Kapalbhati, however, is rather different and is a kriya. *Kapal* means 'skull' and *bhati* means 'furnace'. Kapalbhati cleanses the entire skull, removing all diseases from the head and stimulating the central nervous system.

Method

Sit tall and relaxed in a suitable posture, such as the Padamasana or the Sukasana. Lean slightly forward, breathe in fairly quickly and exhale extremely rapidly and forcefully. Repeat this ten or twelve times without stopping. Concentrate on the exhalation and feel that you are getting rid of all the impurities and toxins. Although the emphasis in this technique is on the out-breath, the amount of air taken in and breathed out is equal. Thus the in-breath is slightly longer and rather gentler. Repeat the whole exercise three times with a few moments pause in between. If you feel giddy and dizzy, stop; close your eyes, and meditate for a few moments. Do not repeat this exercise more than five times in any one day at first.

Note: This exercise should not be practised by people who have high blood pressure.

Tratakam

Tratakam is considered a kriya as it is used to clean the eyes through gazing at an object without blinking. Tears tend to flow and thus the eyes are cleansed. The greater effect which is obtained through Tratakam practice is described later in Chapter 15.

14 Relaxation

It is most important to practise a good relaxation technique after an asana programme for a number of reasons. Firstly, it allows the venous blood to return to the heart, and all the hormones which have been secreted by the endocrine system during the programme to be mixed by the heart. Secondly, the relaxation allows the blocked energy which has been trapped as psychosomatic tension to flow properly through the body. Thirdly, by proper relaxation you will be able to expand beyond your own body image.

Shavasana

Shav means 'the corpse' and whilst the Shavasana may appear extremely easy, it is in fact one of the most advanced postures so far examined.[1]

Method

Lie flat on your back on the ground. Have your feet a little apart and your arms away from the sides of your body, palms facing upwards. Adjust the position of your head so that it is comfortable. Make sure that there is no tension in the back of your neck and you can swallow easily.

In the beginning this posture may not necessarily appear to be one of the most comfortable. This is because of the psychosomatic tensions which you probably have somewhere in your body. Before we go to sleep, we usually manipulate our body, move around, fidget until we get into a suitable position which feels more or less comfortable. In fact this position may be extremely unbalanced, yet we find it comfortable because we are balancing the tensions in our body. This is not real relaxation, but simply like balancing a bucket of water that we are holding in our right hand by holding another bucket of water in the left hand. Our psychosomatic tensions will get no better unless we are able to free them.

Shavasana is potentially the most relaxed and comfortable position of all. If at first you feel tensions anywhere in your body, you know that those are the areas on which you need to work. These are points which have already experienced some kind of disease or damage. It is quite common to feel old wounds and old diseased areas producing a dull ache. This is in fact a good sign as it means that these areas are being completely rebuilt by pranas. This stage of experiencing tensions will quickly pass with proper practice, but sharp and sudden pains are of quite a different nature and you should report them immediately to your teacher. It usually means that you have done something wrong as proper practice of yoga is not painful. As your mind wakes up you may become aware of pains which you might have had for several years but have kept below the thres-

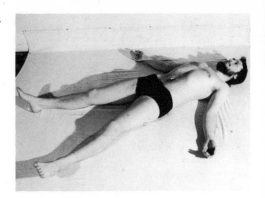

hold of awareness. They are not new pains, you are now experiencing them and recognising them for the first time. Starting Hatha Yoga practice is rather like a city-dweller going for a holiday in the countryside. He breathes fresh air, walks through beautiful landscape, feels unhurried, relaxed and happy. When he returns to the city he feels hemmed in, unable to breathe, dirty and hard-pressed. Everything seems to be in a rush and the city suddenly becomes a pain to him.

There are two ways we can learn—through pain or through awareness. Unfortunately many of us choose pain: yoga chooses awareness. In the beginning students sometimes talk about their friends and relations as though they were changing when, of course, it is not the friends and relations who are changing but the student who is changing through new awareness.

Basic relaxation technique

Lie in the Shavasana, close your eyes and relax. Concentrate first of all on your right big toe; experience it mentally, relax it, let it drift away in consciousness. Do this for the rest of the toes on your right foot, relaxing each in turn. Relax your right foot and ankle, mentally experiencing each part in turn. Relax your calf, your right knee and your right thigh. Completely relax your right leg, feel it grow warm and tingling. Repeat the process exactly for the left leg.

Next relax your buttocks and your pelvic and abdominal muscles. Then relax the entire length of your back and your chest, especially the area around your heart. Now concentrate on your right thumb; experience it and relax it. Relax in turn all the fingers on your right hand. Relax your right wrist, your right forearm, elbow and upper arm. Completely relax your right arm, feel it grow warm and tingling. Repeat the process exactly for the left arm. Next relax your right and left shoulders. Then relax your neck at the back and the sides, your jaw, mouth and tongue. Relax the muscles around your ears, nose and cheeks and then deeply relax your eyes and eyebrows. Relax your forehead and all the muscles leading up to the top of your head. Your entire body should now be relaxed and warm and tingling. Check your body for any tensions and relax them completely.

Notice that the relaxation is done upwards from the feet to the top of the head. This is a different order to certain other kinds of yoga relaxation tech-

niques. By practising this method you will obtain a very deep state
your body tensions will leave you and your body will be rebui
asleep. You may, of course, practise this relaxation technique in
sleep, but after the asana programme the object is to wake you
consciousness.

In the initial stages of practice you may find that parts of your body twitch
irritatingly. For example, your eyes may remain tense and flicker. Only proper
practice will get you past this point, no amount of reading or theory can help
you. Be sensitive to your body, let it teach you its secrets. It will teach you how to
relax, it will show you where you have your tensions and problems and potential
sites of disease. The whole universe is your teacher and your body is no less so.

Do not practise yoga relaxation for too long at a stretch; ten minutes is about
right initially. Students often practise for too long and progress is inhibited by
this. It is better to perfect relaxation in ten minutes than it is to perform a partial relaxation over a longer period. You are liable to lose some of the benefits of
your asana programme by remaining in the Shavasana too long. Naturally, the
relaxation should not be done too quickly.

When you wish to end your relaxation, gradually move your fingers and
slowly touch your face. In this way you will retain the psychological and physiological benefits of the technique. You are throwing away many of the benefits if
you hastily jump up. Come out of the Shavasana carefully and steadily. Retain
the feeling of relaxation and expansion of awareness throughout the rest of your
life.

One problem that sometimes occurs with beginners is disassociation from the
body. It is not uncommon for the student to suddenly find himself looking at his
own body as if from a distance. If it has not happened before it can be a little
disconcerting and even shocking, and the shock is liable to bring one back to the
body with a thump. If this happens do not worry; it is a positive and well-known
occurrence.

The perceptual mind (manomaya kosha) is not completely dependent on the
physical brain and it can be dissociated from the physical body through relaxation. This sometimes happens spontaneously to people who have had no con-
nection with yoga practice. It often happens in highly emotional situations, such
as car accidents. Many people have experienced it and many people will experience it in the future, but there is nothing to fear, it is perfectly natural. When it
happens to you it will be independent proof of the perceptual mind. Most of us
are thoroughly involved in our bodies to the extent that this experience seems
abnormal and weird, although it is just part of waking up to realise that previously you have been hardly living.

Yoga practice will open up a vibrant, exciting, living, fulfilling universe. If
you practise yoga purely in order to obtain experiences, however, you are simply
wasting your time. You will be like the man who believes that money can pur-
chase happiness and so he spends his entire life working hard, doing all the
things he does not like, treading on people and creating enemies in order to

ass a fortune. He achieves that fortune after years of effort, only to find that he is alone without a friend. People only want him for his money, he dislikes himself and despises other people. He has bought unhappiness through ignorance. We are all free to make mistakes but we can learn from others. You can learn quickly or slowly, it does not really matter in cosmic terms. All roads lead to yoga, and while some are long and winding and others are straight and narrow, there is no virtue in arriving there first.

In the New Testament there is a parable about a vineyard keeper who hired men to work in his vineyard and paid them the same amount at the end of the day whether they had worked from the morning, midday or evening.

Yoga Nidra

The relaxation technique described above is one of the fundamental techniques of yoga. It develops into a practice called Yoga Nidra. *Nidra* means 'sleep', and in a state of Yoga Nidra the mind is expanded and illuminated, while the body is asleep.

Method

Practise relaxation in the Shavasana. When you are completely relaxed, concentrate on the top of your head. Use your imagination to help you a little and imagine waves of relaxation entering the top of your head and rippling down over your body, relaxing you completely. With each in-breath imagine the wave entering the top of your head, and with each out-breath imagine the wave of relaxation rippling down through your body. Experience your body melting into a warm ocean of Prana, just as ice melts into water and water in vapour. Feel your body become more deeply and deeply relaxed. Practise for several minutes.

Then concentrate on the region of your heart. Use your imagination to help you and imagine Prana—vibrant bio-energy—moving from your heart to your legs. Feel your toes and legs tingle slightly as it reaches them. Direct the Prana from your legs, back to your heart. Send Prana from your heart to your chest and abdomen, and then experience it returning to your heart. Send Prana from your heart to your arms; experience your hands and arms tingling slightly and then return the Prana to your heart. Now send the Prana from your heart to your head; experience your head growing lighter and vibrant, and then return the Prana from your head to your heart. Then send the Prana from your heart to your entire body; feel your body tingling as it melts into cosmic vibration—Prana. Feel Prana returning to your heart from your whole body. Send Prana from your heart to the ends of the earth and then experience it returning from the four corners of the earth to your heart. Send Prana from your heart to the sun, moon and stars. From the entire universe, experience Prana returning to your heart. Experience the whole universe within you. Experience that all is Self and that there is no separation.

Whilst you are in Yoga Nidra you may specifically recharge and magnetise various areas of your body.

Practical

Place your hands one on top of the other on the centre of your chest, above your heart. Breathe deeply and gently and experience Prana entering your heart from your hands. At first you will feel it as a warmth and later as a pulsating magnetism. After a minute or two place your hands, palms down, on your solar plexus. Experience Prana entering your solar plexus from your hands, recharging it. After a minute place your palms in the same way at the centre of your pelvis. Experience Prana entering your pelvis, charging and magnetising it. After one or two minutes place your hands, palms down, at the base of your throat and then experience Prana entering your throat, recharging it. After one or two minutes place your hands over your eyes, one palm cupped over each eye, and experience Prana entering your eyes as brilliant white light, which may be in sheets or in brilliant flashes. Feel your eyes being recharged and refreshed. Place your hands by your sides, palms upwards. Feel completely refreshed, recreated and expanded.

If you wish you may place your hands one on top of the other, palms down, on any part of your body you specifically wish to recharge. If an area of your body caused you trouble through an accident or disease, this technique will speed up the healing process. Use your imagination to help you. Imagine Prana moving from your heart to the part you are recharging. Feel confident and certain about what you are doing. Know that this technique has been tried out and tested over thousands and thousands of years and that the results are guaranteed. If you do not experience positive results at first, do not be disappointed but go on practising under a good teacher.

Undoubtedly you can achieve any state that has ever been achieved before. Yoga Nidra is a higher state of consciousness. At the moment you may identify with your body and believe that your physical body is your essential Self. In the early stages of Yoga Nidra you will find yourself experiencing things as though they were within you, yet they will be occuring some distance away from your physical body. For example, sounds several feet away will be felt in your body. You will prove to yourself that you are a cosmic entity, omnipresent. As you expand you will find yourself more and more in harmony with the entire universe. As this happens, the basic harmonies and rhythms of the body will settle down as the bio-electricity of your body smooths out into gentle rhythms from its present chaotic buzzing. To observers your body may look asleep however your observers will seem asleep to you.

Pratyhara

With deliberate practice of relaxation and Yoga Nidra you will find that you liberate your psychic energy, which has been invested in your body. You will discover that this energy may be directed at will. Many an apparently impossible task can be performed by this method eg moving objects without touching them, or materialising objects from out of the air. But the yogi is not interested in these tricks; they are of interest only to the worldly minded. These abilities are rarely demonstrated by a true yogi, but by people who have achieved a limited ability and have remained stuck at that stage of attainment. However this psychic energy may be collected and directed for specific work. The yoga technique for doing this is called Pratyhara. The first half of Pratyhara is the withdrawal of energy. Psychic energy may be removed from a part of the body or even from the entire body to produce anaesthesia. The second part of Pratyhara is the application of this energy for the achievement of higher states.

15 Tratakam

In psychology the gaze is known to be most important. The blink-rate of the eye reveals the nervous state of a person. Social dominance and confidence is expressed through eye movement and gaze and emotional changes are clearly seen in the fluctuations in the size of the iris. But in yoga psychology the gaze is even more important. Most of us have tried gazing at the back of a person's neck to make him look round and are so often successful that we are convinced it is the gazing that does it. Again most of us have felt the gaze of someone on the back of our head. In physics we know that gazing directs plasma—ionised gas—which is so different from ordinary gas that it is considered a fourth state of matter. Under controlled experiment it is possible to demonstrate the effect of gazing at a diode bulb. Additional ionisation may be caused in the bulb from a distance causing it to light up and, under conscious control, the bulb may be lighted and turned off at will. Clouds in the sky may be dispersed by staring at them. Until you have done this you may find it difficult to believe. Stare concentratedly at any smallish cloud and you will find that the point you are staring at becomes deep blue and then shortly afterwards the cloud disperses. Similar clouds nearby will not be dispersed. Anyone can learn this ability within a few hours' practice.

Close your eyes for a minute and press your eyeballs hard with your hands, you will find that you see all kinds of geometrical patterns of light. They can be very brilliant and fascinating. What is this light, which cannot have come from outside as your eyes are shut? It is your own light. It is exactly the same light that you see all the time, although normally you project the light out, so that it appears to be outside of yourself. You are a being of light. Your entire body is built of light. This is a scientific truth, not a symbolic mystical statement.

Tratakam is the Sanskrit name given to the practice of training and directing the gaze. It is a high-level concentration technique. Tratakam may also be used as a kriya to clean the eyes, but the practice of Tratakam is far more than this. Through mastering this technique you can learn to control your mental waves, check the restlessness of your mind, and awaken your brain in order to manifest greater consciousness.

Simple Tratakam

Cut out a circular disc of coloured card about 4in across and paste it on to a white sheet of paper. Place it about 6ft in front of you, just a little below your eye-level. Sit in a comfortable position and relax from the top of your head

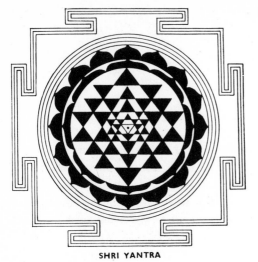

SHRI YANTRA

down, as you would in the Composure. Let all your thoughts go and concentrate for about ten minutes on the disc. Try not to blink, but gradually open your eyes wider and wider to counteract the tendency to blink. Remember that everything you experience is yourself. With a little practice you may see lights of brilliant colour moving around the surface of the disc. You may practise this technique with different coloured discs for different effects. Remain highly alert and aware, do not go into a trance or into a sleepy state. Allow Tratakam to teach you. Practise Tratakam on all kinds of objects: trees in the daylight; the moon at night; your own fingers; your reflection in a mirror. You will discover new worlds of light and colour. Everything has auras, everything is pulsating with energy.

With practice of Tratakam you will learn to see things that are not physically present at the time but have been there in the past or will perhaps be there in the future. Today it is possible to take photographs of things that are not physically present. Although this sounds like science fiction, it is true. Yoga practice will awaken you to many new worlds. Tratakam on a magnet will enable you to see the lines of magnetic energy which surround it. You will be able to test some of your experiences against scientific observation, through the use of infra-red cameras and other detectors. Traditionally Yogis practise Tratakam on the Shri Yantra and this will give you insights into the nature of the universe.

Do not gaze too long—you will find five minutes long enough at first—then close your eyes, place the palms of your hands over them and press gently. You will find this will relieve your eyes of strain.

Special forms of Tratakam are called drishti, of which Nasagra and Bhruma-dhya Drishti are two examples.

Nasagra Drishti

Sit in a suitable posture and relax your body. Have your head tilted a little bit

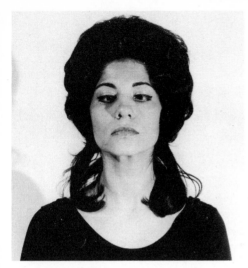

forward, half close your eyes and gaze unblinkingly at the tip of your nose. Practise this for about two minutes at first and then increase it to five minutes or longer as you find it comfortable. After practice, close your eyes and press them gently with the first two fingers of each hand. Blink slowly and deeply and then open your eyes. Blink a little.

You may well perceive new and wonderful smells. This practice works on the cranial nerves which lead back into the brain. It will help improve your memory and the central nervous system as a whole is stimulated. In yoga it is said that you are awakening Kundalini in practising Nasagra Drishti.

Bhrumadhya Drishti

This second drishti should be practised after Nasagra Drishti. Sit in a suitable posture and relax your body from the head down. keeping your spine straight. Concentrate with half-closed eyes on the centre of your forehead, just above and between your eyebrows. Gaze steadily at this point for about two minutes at first. Increase this time to about five minutes later, and after further practice this time may be increased to about about ten minutes or longer. Do not strain your eyes. Close your eyes and place the first two fingers of your hands on your eyes. Breathe deeply and relax. Blink a little.

Through this practice the central and autonomic nervous systems are awakened. This is achieved through stimulation of various cranial nerves which innervate the eyes, nose, face and neck.

Many powers develop through the practice of yoga, be it through a specific technique, such as Tratakam, or through work. These powers must be accepted as part of our omniscient, omnipresent and omnipotent nature. Concentrate on manifesting the highest and do not play games with the phenomena of a lower order, unless you wish to be side-tracked.

There is an interesting story about a yogi who had attained great powers of

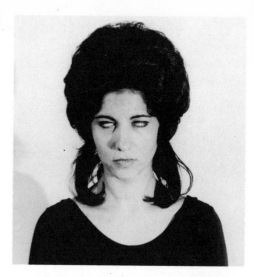

concentration through various disciplined practices. Once a little bird disturbed his meditation and he looked up at this bird with malice in his eyes. The bird fell to the ground, dead. This pseudo-yogi sensed power and became arrogant and dominating. One day, in the course of his wanderings, he came across a house and shouted out, demanding attention (it is the practice in India to treat wandering yogis with hospitality). There was no reply, so he shouted louder, and finally a voice called out asking him to wait a few seconds. He was enraged, and when, after a little while, a woman came to the door the yogi glared at her, but nothing happened. She spoke calmly and serenely to him saying 'See, I am not like the little bird who shrivelled up when you looked at it.' 'How do you know this? It happened many miles away,' questioned the somewhat disillusioned yogi. She replied 'I too have many powers but I have not achieved them through the practices that you have followed. I have these powers because I have faithfully, concentratedly and selflessly served my husband who has been ill and incapacitated for many years.' The yogi learned a great lesson.

16 Meditation

Perhaps the most important of yoga practices is meditation. Meditation, like yoga itself, has both an absolute and a practical definition. Meditation is a state, identical to the state of Yoga, and it is also a practice, which involves the laying aside of the personality in order to experience the state of meditation.

Modern experimental psychology has shown that the perceptual world is an actively constructed world which is projected out. Everything we experience is ourself. However, it is important to understand the difference between the Self as the experiencer and the Self as the experience. In the dualistic world of relativity, the Self is quite distinct from the experience which the Self observes. If we wish to experience ourself then we have merely to let go of everything that is not ourself; and here we have a paradox. There is the Self as the experiencer and also the Self projected out as experience. This leads us to the discovery of the two aspects of meditation.

The one type of meditation is the experience of Self as subject alone, that is, the state of being as against the state of experiencing. This meditation is called Nirguna Samadhi. The other type of meditation is that in which everything is experienced as Self. This is called Saguna Samadhi.

Ancient yoga philosophy and modern experimental psychology agree that what we experience as the world is in fact a partial experience of ourself which is projected out. Thus our experience of the world is not wrong but is illusory if we take it to be a complete picture. When we are experiencing we are living in a partial reality, whereas when we are not experiencing but are being, we are living in absolute reality. This is the experience of Self as it actually, completely and wholly is.

A person who is experiencing the Self as it absolutely is, is said to be liberated, to have achieved Moksha. The yogi who has achieved this state and remains in it all the time, but has also an experience of the projected world as Self, is called a Jivan Mukta. He experiences the world but realises its true nature; he is in the world but not of it, like the lotus which is resting upon the water but is left untouched by it.

The process of meditation is the exact reversal of the process of creation. It is a gradual letting go of the levels of personality in order to be left alone (all one) with the Self. It is because of constant creative effort that we do not normally perceive the true nature of the Self. This creative effort is called Maya in Sanskrit.

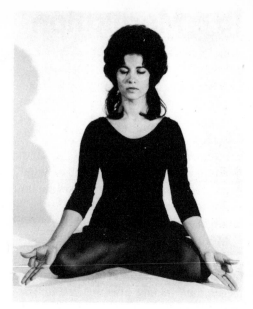

The Stages of Meditation

The stages of yoga, discussed in Chapter 2, form a step-ladder which helps us to mount to the highest state of perfect meditation and thus achieve self-realisation.

The first two stages of yoga, Yama and Niyama, consist of taking hold of ourself and deciding to practise meditation. In many ways the first two stages are the most important as the major difficulty in meditation is actually making the effort to begin practising it. All difficulties after that are far less problematical. The third stage, Asanas, is to sit in a comfortable position and relax the body completely. Normally our body and mind are in constant movement all the time. In order to experience ourself as we really are we must still this constant movement, and so we relax, close our eyes and generally cut out sensation. In the fourth stage, Pranayama, we expand and free our energy in order to get beyond our usual limited identification which blocks the expression of pure consciousness. In the fifth stage, Pratyhara, we collect this energy together in order to overcome the countless years of negative, limiting auto-suggestion which has appeared to enslave our consciousness. At this point we find that long-term memory is our major stumbling-block. It manifests as words, thought and images which enter our mind every few seconds. It is a constant process which most people find impossible to get beyond. Certainly, creative thinking is not possible unless you have the ability to control your thoughts, and this may be tested out by simply attempting to stop thinking. Very few people are able to stop thinking for more than a few seconds at the most. Moreover, there are very few original thinkers in this world. Most thoughts have been programmed into us by advertising, education, indoctrination and social background and contacts.

At the next stage, Dharana, we can overcome the thinking process by introducing an image over and over again to the mind, rather like introducing the
same frame over and over again in a cinema film. As the cinema film would
appear to be still like a slide, so the mind appears to be still, and through this
process we can in fact still the mind. In practice this leads automatically to the
seventh stage, called Dhyana. Dhyana is the total concentration state of pure
awareness and is the technical name for meditation. If Dhyana is maintained
for a long time, the state changes from a temporary concentration to a permanent concentration state and is called Samadhi.

At first it takes three or four days to get into Samadhi, the reason for this
being very simple. The mind is rather like water in that it reflects the Self which
looks into it. Water can be continually agitated by stirring, and in yoga these
'stirrings' or disturbances are known as vitarkas. When we stop stirring, and
this is basically what meditation practice is, the water does not immediately
become still, but takes several minutes to become completely smooth. The mind
too takes a little while before it becomes still, even after the disturbance has
ceased. If the stirring is stopped only for a very short time, then you may not
notice that the mind has begun to slow and settle. The calmness has to be maintained for quite a long time before it becomes obvious that you are achieving
something. When water becomes still, it acts as the perfect mirror to reflect the
Self. When the mind becomes still, the Self is perfectly reflected and this is
called Self-realisation or enlightenment.

Enlightenment is not the same as perfection, but merely the first stage in
achieving it. Perfection is the consolidation of enlightenment and is achieved
when all the long-term memories, known as samskaras in Yoga, are burned up
and discarded.

Practical meditation technique

Meditation should occupy twenty-four hours of every day. Initially, practice may
be divided into two parts—half an hour when one applies the specific meditation
technique and twenty-three and a half hours when one reflects that specific technique.

Sit in a suitable posture, such as the Padmasana. Check that your position is
upright, alert and comfortable and then relax from the top of the head down.
Close your eyes and concentrate on your heart. Practise the Yoga Nidra expansion technique. Collect your energies and direct them from your heart up into
your head and concentrate on the point just above and between your eyebrows.
Now you are ready to practise Dharana.

Perhaps the most effective Dharana technique is Mantra. *Man* means 'thinking' and *tra* means 'protection', and Mantra is a means by which you can protect yourself from, or take yourself beyond, thinking, which prevents you from
experiencing yourself as you wholly are.

The sound 'aum' may be used as an effective mantra, or an alternative is
'ram'. Your teacher will be able to give you a suitable mantra. Repeat your

mantra over and over again mentally, concentrating on it fully. Your teacher may teach you to chant your mantra, and this is a very effective technique indeed. As you repeat your mantra your whole mind, all your mental waves, will become harmonised. Your brain activity will fall into a simple rhythm as you tune in to the Self.

After a few minutes of mantra repetition you will be able to stop as your mind will have become still. This period of perfect silence, complete awareness, when there is neither object of consciousness nor any subject but only an undifferentiated state of being, is meditation.

The experience of Self is not describable in words. It cannot be known to the senses nor can it be conceptualised or imagined. It is beyond conceptualisation or imagination because these are creations of the Self. The pure experience of being, of Self, without the hubbub and buzzing of mental, emotional and physical activity, is the whole purpose of yoga. The experience of Self is described as Satchitananda. *Sat* means 'existence', *chit* means 'consciousness' and ananda can only be described as bliss. When you have given up all action, you are left existing. When you have given up all thinking, you are left aware, conscious. When you have given up all desires, you are left as a state of bliss.

17 The Importance of Food

Our bodies (annamaya kosha) are constructed of the foods we eat. There are three main kinds of solid food which we take into our bodies through our mouths. These are: carbohydrates, which provide most of the energy our body works with; proteins, which are important in building up our body and in growth; and fats, which are the major source of heat for the body. All these foods are derived ultimately from vegetation. Vegetation captures red light from the sun and stores it. It is this red light which is released in the body during the process known as oxidation. Thus our body is constructed of light and our muscles run off red sunlight.

We also take in liquids through our mouths, and the most important of all liquids is water. No life can manifest without water. We take in gases most suitably through the nose. The most important gas for us is oxygen. The manifestation of consciousness depends upon oxygen. Briefly, carbohydrates and other solid foods which have been converted into simple sugars, are broken up by oxygen to release energy and to form carbon dioxide, which is eliminated, and water. The end product of most of the food in our cells is water, which is generally in an ionised state. The oxygen ion is negatively charged and the hydrogen ion is a proton with a positive charge. Life processes are based on proticity.

We also take in, through the nose and to a greater extent through the skin, what is known as plasma. Plasma is considered a fourth state of matter and is basically ionised gas, although it behaves very differently from ordinary gas. These ions depend upon water in the body, and the health of a person rapidly deteriorates if there is a lack of ions, particularly negative ions. Our most important psychic processes are initiated by radiant energy in the form of photons. Almost all our bodily tissues and major organs depend upon light energy, photons, to maintain their rhythmic processes. Light may enter through the skin, but its major entrance is through the eyes.

The last major kind of food is the most important of all, and this is Prana. Prana enters through the medulla oblongata during deep sleep. It is associated with a subtle form of sound called nadam. All food is a form of energy, Prana, and the human body is capable of changing one form of energy into another, for example, physical and chemical energies are transformed into biological and psychological energies.

Suitable Food

In yoga, food is known to have not only a physiological effect but also definite psychological effects. All food is divided into Sattvic, Rajsic or Tamsic food according to its effect on the individual. In the *Bhagavad Gita*[1] it says that the foods which promote life, vitality, strength, health, joy and cheerfulness, which are sweet, soft, nourishing and agreeable, are liked by the Sattvic. The foods which are bitter, sour, saltish, very hot, pungent, harsh and burning, producing grief, pain and disease, are liked by the Rajsic. Food that is spoilt, tasteless, putrid, stale and unclean, is liked by the Tamsic. In the *Hathapradipika*[2] it says that eating pleasant and sweet food after it has been offered to Shiva (that is, it is not taken for ego satisfaction), and leaving a quarter of the stomach empty, is known as Mitahara. Eating food which is bitter, sour, pungent, salty or hot, or eating green vegetables, sour gruel, rancid fermented oil, betel nut, mustard and sesame, fish, meat, yoghurt, milk which has lost its butter, certain grains, oil cakes, asafoetida and garlic, or drinking alcohol, is said to be unwholesome. Food that has been heated up again, is dry, is excessively salty or sour, has gone bad and is indigestable, or has excessive roughage, is unwholesome and should be avoided. The good grains—wheat, rice, barley and particular kinds of good rice—milk, ghee, butter, sugar, candy, honey, dry ginger, cucumber and the five leafy vegetables, kidney beans and water collected when the sun is in Magha (that is a short period which occurs once each month) are considered to be wholesome food for the advanced yogi. The yogi should eat food that is nutritious, sweet and unctious, products of cow's milk and nourishing food of their own choice suitable for practice of yoga.

Fasting

There are a number of reasons for fasting, the least important being to overcome the craving or the desire for food. This is a form of self-discipline called Tapasya. By reducing the amount of solid food intake, the average energy, or the average vibration of the body, may be raised. Biologically, fasting breaks down the protein in the body cells and this has a tonic effect. There are a number of other reasons for fasting, one of which is to remove toxins from the body.[3] Specialist fasts in combination with certain other practices may be used to get rid of certain diseases and other problems.

It is important to coat the stomach after practising asanas and finishing yoga practice. At first some care needs to be taken to ensure a proper diet. As you advance in your yoga practice you will not need to put so much consciousness into food, and your need for solid food will rapidly diminish as you get down to efficient yoga practice. At an advanced state it is possible to go without solid foods altogether. You should be more concerned with what comes out of your mouth than with what goes in. Whilst advanced yogis may practise discrimination in their food choices in order to facilitate what they are doing, they do not discriminate between foods on moral or idealistic grounds as they see *all* as Self.

18 Some Considerations

Before starting to practise Hatha Yoga there are a number of questions you should consider and answer for yourself. First of all, make sure you know why you are taking up the practice of Hatha Yoga. Are you doing it to achieve a healthy body? Are you doing it in order to achieve a healthy mind? Are you doing it in order to improve your concentration or to get rid of psychosomatic tensions? There are countless reasons why people take up Hatha Yoga, and many people fail to get very far because they have not discovered their real aim before starting to practise. Every reason for taking up Hatha Yoga is valid, however, as yoga is essentially a process of self-discovery.

Many changes will occur within you as you start your Hatha Yoga practice. Are you prepared to grow and change? A great many people are not, even though they may say they are. If you are afraid of truth, do not take up yoga. If you are not prepared to practise yoga regularly, do not take it up for you will only waste your own time and that of your teacher and you may well cause yourself harm if you practise in a casual way. Only you can do the work and only you can bear the responsibility for your own actions in life. Your friends will notice you growing and changing and not all of them will understand what is happening to you. If you are practising yoga with a proper attitude nothing bad will befall you, everything will be positive. You will undergo great changes, however, and so sort out your attitudes to yourself, to the world and to people around you before you start. It will save you a lot of problems later on.

When you do start yoga practice there are a number of postures you should not do initially. This will depend on your psychological and physiological state of health. If you have a good teacher he will make sure that you only practise what is good, right and timely for you. If you have a bad teacher then we hope that you will learn enough from this book to realise that some things should not be practised at first and that other things should be taken slowly. We sincerely hope that this book will enhance your practice, but unless you put the methods described in this book into practice, then the whole book will be worthless. Like all the yoga books of the past, it is not intended to replace the teacher. Nothing of real value can be learned from a book, but sometimes a book may help you value real learning.

Yoga teaching is not something that can be learnt in a few years but is a lifetime study and practice. For personality reasons you may not be able to learn from every potential teacher, although as you progress in yoga you should be able to learn from everything and everyone. One of the great problems a student wishing to learn Hatha Yoga practice has, is finding a good teacher. Most students do not know how to recognise a good teacher. Fundamentally, a teacher is a good student and a good teacher is one who is always improving and growing personally. Here are some basic criteria by which you may dismiss the absolute fraud who is pretending to be a yoga teacher.

80-90 per cent of the people in the West do not know precisely where their own heart is. When you ask people to point to their heart, they miss, pointing to their lungs or stomach or elsewhere. Most people are incredibly ignorant about even their own basic anatomy. If a potential teacher does not know where the heart is or where the liver, spleen and kidneys are, then this may be taken as a sign of definite lack of application of knowledge. Most intelligent people can point to the heart or liver in a medical diagram, but they are unable to point to these organs in themselves. If a yoga teacher does not know precisely where the organs of the body are then he is no yoga teacher. It is chronic irresponsibility to teach practices which have effects on the body without at least a basic understanding of what those effects are. It is a yoga teacher's role to know more or less what is going on inside his students. If he does not know he is being irresponsible and no yogi is irresponsible. Find out exactly where your own bodily organs are and you will be able to quickly and easily test a potential yoga teacher.

The second test is based on the fact that no yoga teacher can do his job properly unless he knows you as an individual. The precise effects of an asana depend upon the nature of the person practising them, therefore, if a teacher attempts to teach yoga practices, such as asanas, without first getting to know his students, he is being irresponsible. In India if a student went to a proper yoga teacher it was traditional for him to spend some time, perhaps several years, waiting for the teacher to begin to teach him yoga practices. This delay was necessary for the teacher to get to know the student thoroughly. In most parts of the world today, and particularly in the West, we do not have time to use this procedure. Things have to be speeded up. If you have a teacher who works with you individually then this is best. Make certain in your own mind that your teacher is getting to know you as well as he can. If he is a good teacher he will be able to do it very quickly indeed. He will have ways of seeing into your inner nature and of knowing what is going on inside you. He will be able to answer most of your questions satisfactorily.

If you are one student amongst a large class then your teacher will almost certainly use a questionnaire to help get to know you and gain the essential facts which are required. The teacher needs to know your medical history and to have some kind of idea about your personality as a whole. If your teacher does not use a questionnaire or make some other effort to discover facts about you he is either a super yogi or he is lazy and irresponsible.

The third test is the greatest of all. The only thing a yoga teacher has to offer is himself. If you wish to learn yoga you can only learn it from a person who is himself an example of yoga. In other words look at the person who may become your teacher. Is that person an example of what you wish to become? Does that

170

person represent your ideal of yoga in life? What kind of manifestation does that person have? You can know precisely what kind of person your teacher is by his achievements, by his behaviour, by the influence he has on the universe around him.

The real yoga teacher treats all people equally. As he treats people appropriately, he does not necessarily treat them in the same way. He fears nothing and has his mind always fixed on the Self. He lives life in the light of truth and is a source of illumination and fulfilment for everyone around him.

There are good yoga teachers to be found. There are great yogis alive on earth today, although they are not necessarily the famous ones. If you truly want to achieve the best results then you will be sufficiently motivated to search out a good teacher.

We have discussed the importance of finding a good teacher in some detail because there are many people today pretending to be great teachers who are giving yoga a very bad name. They are not to be taken as examples of yogis. A yogi is a yogi only because he behaves like one and manifests the consciousness of a yogi. A man is not a yogi simply because he says he is, or because he studies yoga.

Many students try to assess their progress when they take up yoga. Although this is basically a waste of time, it is often irresistible to try to find out how far you have gone. There are a number of traditional signs which tell you that you have achieved perfection in Hatha Yoga.[1] They are, slimness (not thinness) of body, a clear resonant voice, freedom from disease, bright eyes and a shining face, control over your hormones and control over your imagination, the ability to control your energy and a continual awareness of the nadam (sound current). However, rather than spend time congratulating yourself on how far you have gone along the road of yoga, it is better to concentrate on finishing the journey. Concentrate on the final point—Self.

As long as you are aware of yourself as an individual ego you have not got to the first stage of yoga. After the first stage your mind is concentrated upon manifesting Self perfectly, and there is no room for self-assessment in the sense of personal congratulation. All your energy is going into positive work, all is Self. There is no point in comparing your progress with that of anyone else in the universe.

19 Yoga in Everyday Life

Do not get the false impression that the yogi is a person who is withdrawn from life. A yogi is rather a great manifester of life and, at best, an example of how life can be lived to obtain fulfilment and bring happiness to everyone around. If you take up yoga practice your life will change and people around you will notice. Whatever you do you will do better and everyone around you will benefit. Do not be put off by reading about and hearing about the countless practices of Hatha and the other branches of yoga. You do not necessarily need to practise any of these techniques. If you feel you need to obtain a healthier body and a more concentrated mind, then there are these specific practices which will help you to achieve this. There are yoga practices which provide for every need you may have; but remember, you are the creator of your own needs. The world has been often compared to a stage. Yoga tells us that we are not only the actor but we are also the director, producer and the script-writer. In fact we also built the stage and own it.

The script of life is that of a learning programme in which we are given simple lessons and then tested. If we get the answers right we go on to the next stage, if not we have to repeat the lesson, perhaps not exactly but we must master that stage before we can go on to the next one. The first question in the script is, 'What is it that you do not know?' Almost all of us ask some routine question trying to find the answer to that first, fundamental question. There is only one thing that cannot be known and that is nothing, the knower, the Self. Just as we look out through our eyes and it is only our own eyes which we cannot see, so the Self, which knows and experiences all things, cannot know itself. When you know that there is only nothing to be known, that is knowledge.

There is a story of a man who was desperately searching for a great yogi who had achieved the secret of all happiness and contentment. The man searched the world over. Throughout the years he searched and searched and finally tracked the yogi down in a lonely Himalayan valley. 'Tell me the secret of contentment and happiness,' the man asked the sage. 'Agree with everything and everyone,' replied the yogi. 'That is ridiculous,' thundered the man, 'I have never heard anything so stupid, so inane, in my life. You are a fool.' 'I agree,' smiled the sage.

The times we live in are very special. Great changes are taking place throughout the entire world. Everything is speeding up, tensions are becoming greater, knowledge is mushrooming and mankind has never been faced with such problems before. In general, individuals are making one of two responses to the world at this stage. They are either hardening themselves, desensitising themselves and becoming even more selfish and cut off from others, or alternatively they are becoming more sensitive, expanding their awareness, sharing their lives, their knowledge, their possessions with others. This positive response is the beginning of a new age of communication, harmony, creativity and happiness. The new age, however, will not be achieved without things getting a lot worse. Mankind is poised on the brink of the greatest evolutionary breakthrough to occur for millions of years. It is the time in which we must all be vigilant, alert and prepared.

Krishna, who represents the magnetic force of cosmic mind, promised that 'whenever "Dharma" wanes, then I will come'. 'Dharma' is the unfailing practice of living your life as well as you can and doing what you believe to be right. The *Bhagavad Gita* is a story about a battle, in which the hero—a man called Arjuna—represents yourself. He finds himself outnumbered and in a very difficult position, but nevertheless, to uphold what is right, he has got to fight. He and his enemies try to enlist the aid of Krishna and his armies; one side is to have Krishna alone and unarmed, the other side is to have his armies. Arjuna chooses Krishna, even though Krishna has said that he will not fight. His enemies choose the armies. Arjuna wavers, realising the apparent hopelessness of his position. Krishna rebukes him for his weakness and then instructs him on yoga philosophy and practice. Through this Arjuna is enlightened; he finds new heart, new strength and faces up to his situation. He realises that he is but the instrument of supreme consciousness. He is totally concentrated on Self and has become the invincible manifester of righteousness. Aum Shanti Shanti Shanti Aum.

References

If not given below, publication details will be found in the Further Reading section.

Chapter 1
1 Andreya Puharich. *Beyond Telepathy*
2 *Bhagavad Gita,* Chap 2, vs 46
3 Swami Chinmayananda. *Kenopanishad,* Book Trust, Chap 2, vs 3
4 Sheila Ostrander and Lyn Schroeder. *Psychic Discoveries Behind the Iron Curtain,* Bantam, Chap 22
5 *Shrimad Bhagavata Mahapurana,* Book 3, discourse 11
6 Sri Aurobindo. *The Secret of the Veda,* Sri Aurobindo Ashram Trust

Chapter 2
1 Frederick and Theodore Barber. 'Yoga, Hypnosis and Self-control of Cardiovascular Functions', *Proceedings, 80th Annual Convention APA,* 1972
   M. V. Bhole and P. V. Karmbelkar. 'Heart Control and Yoga Practice', *Yoga Mimansa,* Vol XIII, no 4 (Jan 1971)
   Elmer Green, Alyce Green and Dale Walters. 'Biofeedback for Mind/Body Self-regulation', Research Dept, The Meninger Foundation, 30 Oct 1972
2 *Hathapradipika,* Chap 2, vs 76

Chapter 4
1 Ramurti Mishra. *Textbook of Yoga Psychology*
2 John Woodroffe. *The Serpent Power,* Dover

Chapter 5
1 Wottgang Huthe. 'Autogenic Training', *Altered States of Consciousness*

Chapter 6
1 M. V. Bhole and P. V. Karmabelkar. 'Heart Control and Yoga Practice', *Yoga Mimansa,* Vol XIII, no 4, p 53-65
2 P. L. Kokajeshtri. *Vasistha Samhita,* Yogakanda

Chapter 12
1 *Hathapradipika*

Chapter 13
1 *Hathapradipika,* Chap 2, vs 21

Chapter 14
1 K. K. Datey. 'Shavasana—a Yogic Excercise in the Management of Hypertension', *Angiology,* 20 (1969), p 325-33

Chapter 17
1 *Bhagavad Gita,* Chap 17, vs 7-10
2 *Hathapradipika,* Chap 1, vs 28
3 Bieler. *Food Is Your Best Medicine*

Chapter 18
1 *Hathapradipika,* Chap 1

Glossary

Adhara nodal point.

Adho under, beneath.

Adi Deva the primeval god, Purush.

Adi Teya offspring of the original one.

Ahimsa non-violence.

Ajna intuitive centre, subcortical chakra.

Akash space, as the mother of form; radiant ether; the state of mind where all mental waves are emptied and radiant ether shines forth.

Akash Vihari the void of space.

Amrit life-promoting fluid; cerebrospinal fluid.

Angustha the big toe, one of the sixteen adharas.

Anhata the source of vibration and movement in the body; unstruck sound.

Annamaya Kosha the physical or food body.

Anshu the superior.

Antar inner.

Apana forces of elimination.

Aparigraha non-hoarding; non-covetous.

Ardha half.

Arjuna the Pandava prince, hero of the *Mahabharata*; represents the archetypal ego.

Aryan one who lives by the power of the word.

Asana postures and exercises to remove communication blocks, to harmonise the personality and bring about a stilling of the mind.

Atha next, now.

Atman the individual, consciousness.

Aum generalised sound of the universe.

Bhadra having suspicious appearance.

Bahya external.

Bandha control.

Basti washing.

Bhagavad Gita part of the *Mahabharata* describing the battle of righteousness against unrighteousness (ego desire).

Bhastrika a bellows; a method of Pranayama.

Bhedana breaking through; a kind of Pranayama.

Bhoomi Sparsh touching the earth.

Bhramari a bee; a type of Pranayama.

Bhrumadhya the centre between the eyebrows.

Bhujangendra the elevation of mind power.

Brahma the creative deity.

Brahman the supreme, one without a second.

Brahmacharya study of the absolute.

Buddhi intellect, wisdom, cosmic intelligence.

Chakra centre.

Chittam mindstuff.

Chandra the moon; receptive, reflective qualities, also; left nostril, and refers to choroid plexus.

Chitra Nadi grey H-shaped part of spinal column.

Daksha right-handed qualities of initiative, dexterity and leadership; name of a king.

Dhauti cleansing of the upper alimentary canal.

Dakshina right-handed.

Deva higher consciousness, entity.

Dhamanis arteries

Dhanur archer.

Dharana fixation of attention.

Dharma righteousness.

Dhatus cells, tissues.

Divya divine.

Drishti gaze, visual insight.

Dvapar Yuga third period of Mahayuga—an age which ended about 5,000 years ago.

Eka one.

Garuda elevated energy which supports the continued functioning of the universe; vehicle of Vishnu; an asana.

Gomamsa the light of life, individual consciousness.

Gomukha enlightening the head.

178

Guru   teacher.

Hal   a plough; an asana by which energy may be reinvested for higher work.

Hatha   the realm of duality.

Hathapradipika   the means by which the world of duality may be transcended to reveal the light of the Self; the title of a famous Yoga text.

Hiran Mey   having the nature of pure gold.

Hridaya   heart.

Indra   the controller of the senses.

Indriyas   the senses.

Ida   the parasympathetic system; the receptive principle.

Ishvarpranidhanani   identification with the entire manifest universe.

Jala   water, fluid.

Jalandhara   the flow of afferent information.

Janusir   reborn in consciousness; an asana.

Jata Veda   the sum total of the Vedas.

Jathar Agni   digestive enzymes and metabolism.

Jihva   individual self equipped with individual psycho-physical mechanism, sometimes symbolised by the tongue.

Jnana   knowledge.

Jnani   one who knows reality.

Jyoti Mey Linga   creative organ of light energy.

Kailash   superior world; mountain home of Shiva.

Kak   a crow.

Kala   epithelial lining.

Kalpa   an age.

Kali   change.

Kapal Bhatti   a kriya which cleans the sinuses and stimulates the central nervous system.

Kapha   mucosal discharge.

Karma   action and reaction.

Karna   ear.

Kevala   liberation.

Khechari   moving in space.

Krouncha   a heron; an asana; a state of consciousness.

Krishna   magnetic force of cosmic mind.

Kriya   action.

Kshana   moment.

Kumbhak   a pot, container; retention of breath in Pranayama.

Kundalini   spiral energy.

Laya   absorbtion.

Linga   creative organ.

Madhya   middle.

Magha   a short period which occurs each month.

Majja   bone marrow.

Manomaya Kosha   the perceptual body.

Matsya   a fish; enlivening; an asana.

Matsyendra   enlivening the mind.

Mitahara   moderation.

Meru   support of the world; the spine.

Moksha   liberation.

Mudha   motion of the body according to psychic energy; body language.

Mula   root, source.

Mukh   mouth

Murccha   a Pranayama technique leading to loss of awareness.

Nabhi   pancreas, also naval.

Nada   sound current; stream of life and consciousness; cosmic and supracosmic rhythmical vibration.

Nadis   channels along which nada passes.

Namah   name, salute.

Namaskar   recognition of the essential Self.

Nasa   nose.

Nasagra   the tip of the nose.

Nataraj   the supreme dance of the universe of vibration and energy.

Nauli   a kriya acting on the metabolic eliminative organs of the body.

Neti   a kriya which stimulates the ciliated lining of the respiratory tract.

Nritya   dance.

Nidra   sleep; one of the five main kinds of modification of chittam.

Nirguna   beyond the gunas.

Niyama   specific positive practices to enable one to manifest the Self perfectly.

Ojas   hormonal force.

Om   alternative spelling of Aum.

Pada   foot, support.

Padma   lotus.

Patanjali   a great scholar and systemiser of yoga philosophy. He also wrote works on medicine and grammar.

Parisarya Nadi Mandalam   the peripheral nervous system.

Parsurama   an incarnation of Vishnu; an avatar.

Paschimotana   an asana stretching the back.

Peshimukhadwayi   diaphragm.

Phuphusa   lung.

Pingala   sympathetic nervous system.

Plijha   spleen.

Prana   energy; (esp) bio-energy; energy governing incorporation of substances into the body.

Prana Maya Kosha   Pranic or bioenergetic body.

Pranayama   control and expansion of energy.

Pranava   aum.

Pratyhara   withdrawal of psychic energy.

Purakh   controlled inspiration.

Puranas   ancient textbooks on all aspects of life and science. Traditionally there are at least 400,000 of them.

Raja   supreme.

Rajaguna   energetic/emotional quality, electronic force.

Rajakapot   an asana.

Rakta   blood.

Rama   an incarnation of Vishnu; an avatar.

Rajsic   having the quality of rajaguna.

Rasa   plasma, lymph fluid.

Rasana   the taster of experience.

Rechakh   researcher.

Rishi   researcher.

Rupa   form, beauty.

Saguna   with the gunas.

Sahasram   the highest psychic centre in the body.

Samadhi   complete absorption, yoga.

Samana   bio-energy responsible for metabolic processes.

Samskara   memory trace.

Sanskrit   exact, mathematical language.

Santosh   contentment.

Satya   truth.

Saucha   cleanliness.

Sankalpa   synthesis, formitive will.

Sat Chit Ananda   state of existence, consciousness, bliss.

Sarvanga   asana affecting the entire body.

Shakti   force.

Shankini   the fourth ventricle.

Shiva   entity responsible for dissolution of universe.

Siddhi   attainment, power.

Siras   veins.

Sirobalam   the seat of balance, the cerebellum.

Sirobrahman   the seat of consciousness, the cerebrum.

Sirshasana   asana predominantly working on the brain centres.

Sirskam   the medulla oblongata.

Sironadi   cranial nerves.

Smriti   memory.

Somamandalam   pituitary gland.

Srotamsi   capillaries.

Srotas   lymphatic vessels.

Sruti   revealed knowledge.

Sunyadesh   the third ventricle.

Surya   right nostril.

Sushumna   the central nervous system.

Sushumna Kandam   spinal cord.

Svadhiyaya   study of science and literature.

Svadisthana   centre of personal/social energy.

Svarupa   inherent form.

Tamoguna   inertia force.

Tandava   cosmic dance.

Tantra   interwoven.

Tapa   self-discipline.

Tapasya   the practice of Tapa.

Tratakam   meditation with eyes open.

Treeta   the second era of the Mahayuga.

Trikona   triangle.

Triveni   the place where three rivers meet, the hypothalamus.

Udana   bio-energetic force by which sounds are produced.

Upanishad   textbooks of Vedanta.

Ushtra   an asana.

Uddiyana   producing a 'flying up' of energy.

Ujjayi   superior Pranayama technique.

Ushra Svarupa   the embodiment of warmth and life energy.

Uttara Basti   kriya washing the bowels.

Uttitha   raised.

Vajra   radiant energy; an asana.

Vajra Nadi   white part of spinal cord.

Vatnya   gas remover; an asana.

Veda   four ancient textbooks of knowledge—the Rigveda, Yajurveda, Samveda, Athurveda.

Viparita   inverted.

Virabhadra   an asana.

Vishnu   the all-pervading entity responsible for communication and maintenance of the universe.

Vishva   the universe.

Vishuddhi   centre at the level of the throat.

Vitarka   destructive instinctual drives.

Viveka   discrimination between consciousness and matter.

Viyana   bio-energy which controls contraction and expansion of cardiovascular system.

Vrikkau   kidney.

Wama   left side.

Yama   limitation.

Yoga   oneness, unity, perfect.

Yoganushasnam   explanation of yoga.

Yuga   age; era.

Yoni   cosmic receptive organ.

Further Reading

This list is composed of works which the authors have found useful in their practice of Svadhiyaya (study). Books are more or less useless in yoga practice except when they help us to understand and communicate our experience.

The following books are on various aspects of yoga philosophy, and if the student concentrates receptively whilst reading them, their authors can come through the words.

Bhagavad Gita, trans Radhakrishnan, Allen & Unwin, 1948
Feurstein, George, and Miller, Jeanine. *A Reappraisal of Yoga,* Rider (New York)
Mahabharata, Bharatiya Vidya Bhavan
Mishra, Ramurti. *Textbook of Yoga Psychology,* Lyrebird Press, 1963
Osborne, Arthur (ed). *The Collected Works of Ramana Maharshi,* Rider (New York)
———. *The Teachings of Ramana Maharshi,* Rider (New York)
Radhakrishnan. *The Principal Upanishads,* Allen & Unwin, 1953
Shrimad Bhagawat Mahapurana, trans G. L. Goswami, Gita Press
Sri Ramcharitmanasa, Gita Press
Woodroffe, John. *The Serpent Power,* Ganesh, 1972
———. *The World As Power,* Vedanata Press (Holywood: CA)

There are countless books about yoga and yoga practice. These three between them cover a great deal of traditional ground. Remember that, like our own, these are an accessory to a good teacher and cannot replace him.

Hathapradipika, trans and commentary Kevin and Venika Kingsland, Penguin Books (UK)
Iyengar, B.K.S. *Light on Yoga,* Allen & Unwin, 1968
Mishra, Ramurti. *Fundamentals of Yoga,* Lyrebird Press, 1959

Perhaps the most fruitful area of reading is in science. Yoga practice is founded on science, and the greater the understanding of modern science, the greater the understanding of yoga. The rishis of yesterday are the great scientists of today. Make sure, however, that your reading material is up to date as there has been a major revolution in scientific understanding in the last few years. These books compose a useful introduction:

Andrews, D. H. *Symphony of Life,* Unity Press, 1966

Asimov, Isaac. *The Human Body,* New American Library (New York), 1964
———. *The Human Brain,* Houghton Mifflin (Boston:Mass), 1964
Bieler. *Food Is Your Best Medicine,* Neville Spearman, 1968
Lewin, Roger. *Hormones—Chemical Communicators,* Geoffrey Chapman
Lewis, J. G. *The Endocrine System,* Penguin Library of Nursing, 1973
Luce, Gay Gaer. *Body Time,* Pantheon (New York), 1971
Ornstein, Robert E. *The Psychology of Consciousness,* W. H. Freeman
Reiser, Oliver. *Cosmic Humanism,* Schenkman, 1966

The following books take the keen student a little further but require a more developed Dharana ability:

Grossman, S. P. *A Textbook of Physiological Psychology,* Wiley (New York), 1967
Ornstein, Robert E. (ed). *The Nature of Human Consciousness,* W. H. Freeman
Puharich, Andreya. *Beyond Telepathy,* Darton, Longman & Todd, 1962
Selkurt, Edward (ed). *Physiology,* Little, Brown (Boston: Mass), 1966, Churchill Livingstone (Edinburgh), 1971
Tart, Charles E. (ed). *Altered States of Consciousness,* Wiley (New York), 1969
Williams, R. H. (ed). *Textbook of Endocrinology,* 4th ed, Saunders
Woodburne, Lloyd S. *The Neural Basis of Behaviour,* Charles E. Merrill (Ontario), 1967

Important articles which are relevant to the yogic quest for understanding can be found scattered through countless journals and textbooks. For example, *Scientific American and New Scientist* often contain valuable material. These four journals are particularly relevant:

The Introquest Letter, Centre for Human Communication, Davidsonville, MD
Energy and Character, Abbotsbury Publications, Abbotsbury, Dorset
The Journal of Transpersonal Psychology, PO Box 437, Stanford, California
Yoga Mimansa, Kaivalyadham, Lonavala (near Poona), India

The above lists are neither exclusive nor fully comprehensive, and are offered only as a starting point. The student should actively seek out relevant material and advice from those around him who already manifest a greater understanding.

Acknowledgments

Special thanks must be given to Peter Cox for taking all the photographs in this book and to Pat Baker who did a great deal of its typing in its original form. David Pike gave important feedback and many others contributed in yogic ways by relieving us of other work so that we could write.

We are grateful to the following for the use of the diagrams listed below:

The innervation of the skin: after J. J. Keegan and F. D. Garrett, *Anat. Rec.* 1948

The nervous system: Russell T. Woodburne, *Essentials of Human Anatomy,* Merrill

The spinal cord: Russell T. Woodburne, *Essentials of Human Anatomy,* Merrill

The autonomic system: Russell T. Woodburne, *Essentials of Human Anatomy,* Merrill

The autonomic ganglia and plexuses: Woerdeman, M. W., *Atlas of Human Anatomy*

The cranial nerves: after Frank H. Netter, *The CIBA Collection of Medical Illustrations*

The lymphatic system: *Scientific American,* July 1973

Index

Abdominal: disorder, 136, 150; fat reduction, 107, 108; muscles, 85, 104, 145; organs, 95, 105, 106, 113, 122; pains 79
Aching ears, 97
Acromegaly, 54
Adharas, 34, 120
Adhobasti, 149, 150
Adi deva, 86
Adi teya, 87
Adrenals, 54, 102, 110, *90*
Adrenergic, 39, 74
Ahimsa, 28, 29, 94
Ajna Chakra, 46, 100
Akasha, 64
Akash Vihari, 87
Alimentary, 89, 136
Alternate nostril breathing, 141
Alveoli, 73
Amrit, 58, 118
Amrit Svarupa, 87
Anaesthesia, 158
Anal muscles, 135
Angusthasana, 121, *120*
Anhata Chakra, 39, 58, 108, 110, 116
Anjana, 123
Anjaneyasana, 123
Ankles, 94, 95, 118, 123
Annamayakosh, 72, 167
Antar Kumbhak, 64
Anxiety, 50
Aorta, 67
Apana, 65, 69, 135
Aparigraha, 31
Ardha Matsyendra, 114
Arteries, 67
Arterioles, 67, 68
Arthritis, 42, 89
Arjuna, 173
Asanas, 25, 79, 153, 155, 164, 170; *88-127* programme, 90
Ashtanga position, 83
Ashtanga Yoga, 20, 21
Asteya, 29, 30
Asthma, 97
Aswini Mudra, 149, *132*
Athletics, 88, 91
Atom, 34, 64
Autonomic nervous system, 37, 38, 39, 68, 104, 113, 132, 133, 135, 141, 142, 161
Autosuggestion, 164
Aum, 29, 45, 106

Back ache relief, 108
Back muscles, 105, 107
Backward bending, 90
Bacteria, 70, 72
Bahya Kumbhak, 64

Balance improved, 118
Bandha Janusir, 103
Bandhas, 91, 94, 145, *135-139*
Basti, 147, *149-150*
Bhadrasana, 93
Bhagavad Gita, 16, 168, 173
Bhakti Yoga, 16, 17
Bhastrika, 140, 152, *144*
Bhoomi Sparsh Mudra, *134*
Bhrumadhya Drishti, 160, *161*
Bhujangasana, 104, 105
Bhujangendrasana, 106
Biliousness, 143, 144
Bioelectricity, 157
Bioenergetic: body, 146; effects, 103; feedback, 102; pathways, 146
Bioenergy, 64
Biological: clock, 53, rhythms, 89
Bindu, 121
Blink rate, 159
Blood, 66, 67, 69-70; magnetic properties, 69; clotting, 70
Blood/brain barrier, 72
Blood circulation, 79, 110; aided to legs, 105
Blood pressure, 60, 75, 97, 109, 142, 143, 152
Body image, 153
Body language, 128
Bone marrow, 69, 70, 72
Bones, 89
Brahma, 96, 140
Brahma Bandha, 137
Brahmacharya, 30, 31
Brahma Mudra, 128
Brahman, 11, 86, 138; cave of, 133; breath of, 21
Brahma Nadi, 48
Brahmari, 140, *145*
Brain, 19, 25, 44, 73, 155; activity in mantra, 166; enlivening, 113
Brainwaves, 50
Breathing, 64; rate, 74, 143
Bronchi, 73
Bronchioles, 73
Buddha, 134

Calf muscles, 120
Calcification, 100
Cancer, 58
Capillaries, 67, 68
Carbohydrates, 167
Carbon dioxide, 66, 70, 74, 167
Carotid: artery, 101, 103, 130, 137; nerve, 130; sinus, 68, 109, 137
Catering Yoga, 21
Cells, 52, 64, 66, 67
Central nervous system, 47, 74, 133, 136; programming, 141; stimulating, 88, 131, 145, 161

Cerebellum, control, 120
Cerebral: aqueduct, 47; cortex, 47; hemispheres, 47
Cerebrospinal canal, 47
Cerebrospinal fluid, 74, 113, 134, 139, *55-58*
Cerebrum, 47; frontal lobes, 47; parietal lobes, 47;
   occipetal lobes, 47; temporal lobes, 47
Chakra, definition, 110
Chakras, work on, 88, 89
Chakrasana, 110
Chakra system, 64; traditional, 34-35
Chandra, 48, 113, 134
Chandrasana, 116
Chest, 100
Chin lock, 98
Chitra Nadi, 48
Cholinergia, 143
Cholinergic, 74
Choroid plexus, 47, 134
Ciliated epithelial, 73
Circadian rhythm, 79
Circulatory system, 65, 66, 89
Cloud dispersing, 159
Coccygeal nerve, 118
Colour, 78, 160
Complementary asanas, 90
Complex exercises, 91
Complexion, 100
Communication, 32, 65, 69, 173; blocks, 88, 140
Composure, 80, 160
Concentration, 141, 165; in asanas, 78, 89, 95
Congested liver, 97
Congested spleen, 97
Consciousness, 10, 33, 47, 64, 81, 87, 133, 155, 159,
   173
Constipation, 57, 97, 98, 101, 111, 113, 117, 130, 133,
   136
Crainial nerves, 46, 125, 132, 138, 161
Creation, 21

Daksha, 119
Dakashinanauli, 150
Deep sleep, 50
Dehydration, 72
Desires, 77
Dhamanis, 67
Dhanurasana, 106
Dharana, 26, 139, 146, 165
Dhatus, 67
Dhauti, 147, 149
Dhyana, 165
Diabetes Mellitus, 60, 89
Diabetes Insipidus, 54
Diaphragm, 74
Digestion, improved, 143, 144, 145, 150
Digestive system, 101, 107, 130, 136; troubles, 111
Disassociation, 155
Discipline, 24
Discrimination, 15
Disease, 65; of joints, 108
Displaced uterus, 98
Divya Svarupa, 87
DNA, 20, 37
Drishti, 94, 160
Drugs, 19, 78, 146
Dvaparyuga, 21, 22
Dyspepsia, 97, 98, 113

Earth's pranic fields, 134
EEG, 50, 61, 131
Ego, 11, 16, 17, 23, 24, 30, 33, 58, 65, 138, 171

Eka Pada Angusthasana, 120
Eka Pada Rajakapotasana, 110
Electricity, 72
Electromagnetic: effects, 89; influences, 139; pulses, 68
Electron, 11
Enema, 150
Endocrine system, 52, 72, 88, *37-47*; secretions, 31;
   work on, 88, 97, 106, 153
Enlightenment, 32, 165
Entropy, 64
Environment, 77, 78
Erithrocytes, 70
Eustachian canals, 137
Evolution, 87
Expectancy, 76
Experimental psychology, 163
Eyes, 143; muscles of, 126
Eye and neck exercises, 93, 126

Facial muscles, 128
False identification, 88
Faraday, 11
Fasting, 168
Fat hips, reduction of, 123
Fats, 167
Fever, 143, 144
Fingers, 125
Flatulence, 122
Food, 79, 168
Forward bending, 90
Front of legs, 107

Gandhi, 31
Gastro-intestinal disorders, 98, 149
Garudhasana, 90, *118*
Gaze, 159
Genital disorders, 150
Glottis, closure of, 137
Glycogen, 39, 60
Goblet cells, 73
God, 96
Goitre, 41
Gomukhasana, 70, 100
Gonads, 62, 90, 110, 112, 118
Grand mal, 131
Gravity, 64; effects of, 97, 98
Guru, 77

Haemoglobin, 69, 70
Halasana, 105, *108*
Hamstrings, 86, 101, 102, 117, 124
Hatha, 49
Hathapradipika, 26, 92, 94, 106, 113, 133, 134, 140,
   147, 168
Hatha Yoga, 14, 26, 31, 76, 79, 88, 112, 119, 169,
   170; achievement, 116; mastery, 89; practice, 154;
   programme, 84; signs of progress, 171
Headaches, 89, 99, 152
Headstand, 90
Health, 65
Hearing improved, 125
Heart, 66, 68, 170; rate, 68, 109
Hernia, 97, 98
Hiran Mey, 87
Hormones, 69, 52, 153; adrenalin, 60; androgen, 60;
   antidiuretic, 90; corticotrophin, 54; glucagon, 59;
   hydrocortisone, 60; insulin, 60; melatonin, 53;
   noradrenalin, 60; oestrogen, 60; progesterone, 63;
   somatotrophin, 54; suitability of, 139, thyrotrophin,
   54, thyroxine, 57

188

Hydrogen ions, 70, 74, 167
Hyperinsulinism, 60
Hyperparathyroidism, 57
Hyperthyroidism, 57
Hypnosis, 88
Hypoparathyroidism, 57
Hypothalamus, 46-47, 73, 133
Hypothyroidism, 57

Ida, 46, 133
Illusion, 23
Imagination, 18, 19, 20, 76, 171
Immune system, 72
Indriyas, 92
Insomnia, 145
Intercostal muscles, 116
Intestinal disorders, 150
Ions: potassium, 68; sodium, 68; air, 74, 75
Ishvarapranidhanani, 33
Islets of Langerhans, 59

Jalandharabandha, 146, *137*
Jalaneti, 151
Janusirasana, 70, 102
Jata Veda, 86
Jihvabandha, 138
Jivan Mukti, 163
Jnana Mudra, 94, *134*
Jnana Yoga, 15, 16
Jnani, 15
Joints, 89
Jyoti Mey Lingha, 86

Kakasana, 121
Kala, 73, 115
Kaliyuga, 21, 22
Kalpa, 21
Kapal Bhati, 147, *152*
Kapha, 73, 122
Karma, 14, 133
Karma Yoga, 13, 14
Karnabasti, 149
Kartikeya, 124
Kevali Kumbhak, 140
Khechari Mudra, 133
Kidney, 60, 69, 72, 102, 113
Knees, 94, 95, 118, 123
Krishna, 173
Kriyas, 80, 91, 136, *147-152*
Krounchasana, 124
Kshana, 133
Kumbhak, 64, 140, 142, 143, 144, 145, 146
Kundalini, 19, 20, 104; awakening, 141, 161; and
    mudras, 128, rousing, 113; turning on, 106

Lacteals, 72
Laksman, 123
Lateral ventricles, 47
Laya, 20
Left/right differences in body, 91
Leg muscles, 124
Leucocytes, 70
Light, 10, 12, 15, 29, 53, 81, 86, 100, 159, 167;
    infrared, 11; ultraviolet, 11
Linga, 34, 86
Liver, 59, 69, 113, 143, 144, 145
Long-short eye sight, 126
Love, 17, 20
Lungs, 69, 73; capacity, 74, 85

Lymph, 70, 72; nodes, 72
Lymphatic system, 66, 70-72
Lymphatic vessels, 72
Lymphocytes, 58, 72

Madya Nauli, 150
Magnetic field, 11, 69; energy, 160
Magnetizing brain, 101; body, 156-157
Mahabandha, 130
Mahamudra, 130
Maha Vishnu, 87
Manipura Chakra, 39, 59, 104, 105, 106, 107, 112, *42*
Manomayakosh, 155
Mantra, 18, 86; in postures, 89, 165
Mantra Yoga, 17, 18
Mat, 79
Materializing objects, 157
Matsyasana, 90, 98, 99-100
Matsyendra, 112
Maya, 11, 23, 163
Meditation, 61, 134, 163-166; in padmasana, 95
Medulla oblongata, 55, 58, 74, 139
Menstrual cycle, 62
Metabolism, 106, 150
Mitahara, 94, 168
Moksha, 163
Mount Kailash, 119
Morphine, 76
Mouth, 73
Mucus, 73; membranes, 147
Mudra, 86, 91, *128-134*
Mulabandha, 144, 145, *135*
Murccha, 140, *145*
Muscles, 89

Nabhi, 59
Nada, 106, 137, 138, 171
Nadabandha, 132, *137*
Nadis, 89, 116, 140, 146
Nasagra Drishti, 160
Nasal catarrh, 97
Nasopharyngeal cavity, 141
Natarajasana, 119
Nath School, 112
Nauli, 136, 147, 148, *150*
Neck, 100, 125
Nervous system, 51, 65, 72, 81, 88, 97, 104, 117, 152
Nervous tension, 88
Neti, 147, *151*
Netrabasti, 149
Neurasthania, 97
New Testament, 156
Niyama, 24, 31-33, 94, 164
Nostrils, 73, 74
Nuclear force, 64

Octave, 34
Ojas, 135
Order of a programme, 90
Orgasm, 20
Orgastic potential, 135
Ova, 62
Ovaries, 62
Ovulation, 62
Oxygen, 68, 167

Pacemaker, 68
Padhastasana, 117
Padmasana, 80, 95, 100, 130, 131, 135, 152, 165

Pancreas, 59, 90, 145
Parathyroids, 56, 98, 100, 108, 110
Parvati, 112
Parsurama, 124
Paschimotanasana, 101
Patanjali, 34
Pelvis, 105, 119, 121, 133
Peptic ulcers, 89
Perception—sharpening, 104
Perceptual mind, 155
Perceptual world, 163
Periods, 79
Personality, 12, 23, 48, 64, 88, 97, 122, 137, 169, 170; and stiffness, 91
Perspiration, 142
Piles, 133
Pineal, 90, 97, 100, *37-38*
Pingala, 36, 39, 133
Pin-hole camera, 10
Pitta, 122
Pituitary gland, 90, 97, 100, *38-40*
Plasma blood, 69
Plasma—ions, 159, 167
Platelets, 70
Pleura, 74
Pollution, 31
Pons, 45
Powers, 161
Prana, 25, 34, 64, 68, 69, 72, 74, 103, 156, directing, 89
Pranamaya Kosh, 146
Pranayama, 25, 39, 59, 65, 70, 92, 95, 137, 164, *140-146*
Pranic effects, 89; healing, 146
Pratyhara, 26, 158, 164, *157*
Pregnancy, 79, 150
Preparation, 79
Prodigal son, 87
Prolapse, 133
Proteins, 167
Proticity, 70, 74, 167
Proton, 70
Psi-plasma field, 11
Psychokinesis, 146
Psycho-sexual energy, 108, 121, 135
Psychosomatic energy, 85
Psychosomatic tensions, 14, 81, 88, 89, 91, 94, 101, 117, 122, 124, 153, 169; in small of back, pelvis and front of legs, 106
Puharich, 11
Pulmonary circulation, 66
Purak, 64, 140, 142, 143, 145
Puranas, 22
Purush, 86
Pyloric sphincter, 149

Rajagunarupa, 87
Raja Yoga, 18, 26
Rajoguna, 96
Rajsic, 168
Rama, 123
Rechak, 65, 140, 142, 143, 145, 146
Rectum, 149
Relaxation, 155-158
Reproductive system benefitted, 111
Respiratory system, 65; tract, 66, 73
Reticular activating system, 45
Reticular formation, 45
Rishis, 134

Sahasaram, 97, 117
Salabasana, 104
Samadhi, 26, 27, 165; Saguna, 27, 163; Nirguna, 27, 163
Samana, 65
Samskars, 14, 165
Sankalpa, 80
Sanskrit, 22
Santosha, 32
Sarvangasana, 90, 97, 105, 120
Satchitananda, 166
Sati, 119
Sattvaguna, 96
Sattvic, 168
Satyama, 29
Satyayuga, 21, 22
Saucha, 31-32
Schizophrenia, 61
Sciatic nerves stimulated, 121
Sciatica, 124
Self, 10, 11, 15, 17, 18, 20, 21, 23, 24, 26, 27, 30, 32, 65, 77, 78, 81, 86, 87, 121, 163, 166, 168, 171, 172
Self realization, 165
Sex, 20, 30
Sexual apparatus, rejuvenation of, 110
Sexual debility, 118
Sexual energy, 118, 135
Sexual organs, 98; and psychic energy, 135
Shakti, 20
Shankini, 44
Shatkarmas, 147
Shatkarmasangraha, 91
Shavasana, 153
Shiva, 112, 119, 168
Shoulder, 108, 110, 113
Shri Yantra, 160
Siddhasana, 94, 135
Simbhasana, 125
Simple Pranayama, 140
Sinuses: nasal, 73, 141, 142, 145; diseased, 152
Siras, 67
Sirobalam, 44
Sirobrahman, 47
Sirshasana, 90, 96; dangers, 96
Sitali, 140, *143*
Sitkari, 140, *143*
Skin, 11, 48, 72, 74, 167
Sleep, 50
Small intestine, 72
Smriti, 22
Soft palate, 138
Space, 10, 11, 64
Spermatozoa, 45
Spinal cord/nerves, 39-40, 117, 130, 139
Spine, 81, 85, 88, 104, 108, 110, 111, 113, 117, 119, coccygeal, 94; sacral, 39-40, 101, 102, 106, 117; lumbar, 39-40, 86, 94, 104, 106, 107, 110, 112; thoracic, 39-40; cervical, 48, 100, 109, 110
Spleen, 72, 113, 144, 145
Srotamsi, 67
Srotas, 72
Sruti, 22
Stages of Yoga, 23
Standing balances, 90
Stomach, 40, 149, 168; gas alleviation, 107
Stomach fat, 112
Subclavian vein, 72
Suggestion, 88
Sukhasana, 80, 92, 135, 152

Sun, 70, 81
Sunya Desh, 47
Superior thyroid artery, 98
Suptavajrasana, 109
Surya, 39
Surya Bhedana, 140, *141*
Surya Namaskar, 81-87
Sushumna, 46, 133, 136
Svadisthana Chakra, 39, 101, 102, 110, 117
Svadiyaya, 32
Systematic circulation, 66

Tamoguna, 96
Tamsic, 168
Tandava Nritya, 119
Tantra Yoga, 18, 19, 20
Tapasya, 32, 168
Teacher, 170
Temperature, 79
Testes, 45
Thalamus, 46
Thighs, 94, 121
Thinking, 76
Third ventricle, 133
Thirst, 143
Thoracic duct, 72
Throbocytes, 70
Thymus, 58, 72, 110, 116
Thyroid, 56, 89, 90, 98, 100, 108, 110
Timing, 79; in postures, 89
Tongue roof of, 125
Tonic effect on muscles, 88
Tonsils, 72
Tratakam, 94, 147, 152, *159*
Treetayuga, 21, 22
Trikonasana, 115
Trust, 29
Truth, 29, 78, 171
Twisting, 90, 91

Udana, 65
Uddiyana bandha, 148, *136*

Ujjayi, 131, 140, 145, *142*
Unconsciousness, 87
Upanishads, 22
Ushra Svarupa, 87
Ushtrasana, 112
Uttarbasti, 149
Uttithar Kumarasana, 125

Vagus nerve, 40, 68
Vajrasana, 92, 100, 109, 120, 125, 126
Varicose veins, 98
Vat, 122
Vatnyasana, 122, 133
Vedas, 22
Veins, 67
Venous blood, 74, 153
Venules, 67
Vibration, 64, 65, 119, 137
Viparita Karni, 133, *138*
Virabhadrasana, 122
Visceratosis, 97
Vishnu, 96, 118, 123
Vishvasara Tantra, 35
Vishuddhi Chakra, 56, 98, 100, 108, 110
Vitarka, 24
Viveka, 15, 23
Vyana, 65, 69

Waist—trimming, 116, 117
Wama Nauli, 150
Water, 70, 72, 165, 167
Weak: eye capillaries, 97; heart, 97; interactions, 64
Wrists, 121

Yama, 77, 94, 164, *24-31*
Yoga: definition of, 10, 13, 25, 65, 88, 134; medicine, 91; Mudra, 130; Nidra, 72, *156*; philosophy, 163; progress in, 77
Yogini, 31
Yogipatni, 31
Yoni Mudra, 131, 137
Yuga, 21